Minimally Invasive Procedures in Facial Plastic Surgery

Editor

THEDA C. KONTIS

FACIAL PLASTIC SURGERY CLINICS OF NORTH AMERICA

www.facialplastic.theclinics.com

Consulting Editor

J. REGAN THOMAS

May 2013 • Volume 21 • Number 2

ELSEVIER

1600 John F. Kennedy Boulevard • Suite 1800 • Philadelphia, Pennsylvania, 19103-2899

http://www.theclinics.com

FACIAL PLASTIC SURGERY CLINICS OF NORTH AMERICA Volume 21, Number 2
May 2013 ISSN 1064-7406, ISBN 978-1-4557-7087-8

Editor: Joanne Husovski

Facial Plastic Surgery Clinics of North America (ISSN 1064-7406) is published quarterly by Elsevier Inc., 360 Park Avenue South, New York, NY 10010-1710. Months of issue are February, May, August, and November. Business and Editorial Offices: 1600 John F. Kennedy Blvd., Suite 1800, Philadelphia, PA 19103-2899. Periodicals postage paid at New York, NY, and additional mailing offices. Subscription prices are $373.00 per year (US individuals), $526.00 per year (US institutions), $425.00 per year (Canadian individuals), $628.00 per year (Canadian institutions), $509.00 per year (foreign individuals), $628.00 per year (foreign institutions), $153.00 per year (US students), and $245.00 per year (foreign students). Foreign air speed delivery is included in all *Clinics* subscription prices. All prices are subject to change without notice. POSTMASTER: Send address changes to *Facial Plastic Surgery Clinics*, Elsevier Health Sciences Division, Subscription Customer Service, 3251 Riverport Lane, Maryland Heights, MO 63043. **Customer service: 1-800-654-2452 (US and Canada); 1-314-447-8871 (outside US and Canada); Fax: 314-447-8029; E-mail:journalscustomerservice-usa@elsevier.com (for print support); journalsonline support-usa@elsevier.com (for online support).**

Reprints. For copies of 100 or more of articles in this publication, please contact the Commercial Reprints Department, Elsevier Inc., 360 Park Avenue South, New York, NY 10010-1710. Tel.: 212-633-3812; Fax: 212-462-1935; E-mail: reprints@elsevier.com.

Facial Plastic Surgery Clinics of North America is covered in *MEDLINE/PubMed (Index Medicus)*.

Printed and bound by CPI Group (UK) Ltd, Croydon, CR0 4YY

Transferred to digital print 2012

Contributors

CONSULTING EDITOR

J. REGAN THOMAS, MD, FACS
Professor and Chairman, Department of
Otolaryngology, University of Illinois at
Chicago, Chicago, Illinois

EDITOR

THEDA C. KONTIS, MD, FACS
Assistant Professor, Department of
Otolaryngology-Head and Neck Surgery,
Johns Hopkins Medical Institutions, Facial
Plastic Surgicenter, LLC, Baltimore, Maryland

AUTHORS

JOHN P. ARKINS, BS
Department of Aesthetic Research, DeNova
Research, Chicago, Illinois

WILLIAM J. BINDER, MD, FACS
Assistant Clinical Professor, Department of
Head and Neck Surgery, University of
California, Los Angeles, Beverly Hills, California

EDWARD D. BUCKINGHAM, MD
Director, Buckingham Center for Facial Plastic
Surgery, PA, Austin, Texas

SCOTT R. CHAIET, MD
Facial Plastic and Reconstructive Surgery,
Williams' Center of Plastic Surgery Specialists,
Latham, New York; Clinical Instructor, Division
of Otolaryngology-Head and Neck Surgery,
Department of Surgery, Albany Medical
Center, Albany, New York

RAHMAN CHAUDHRY, MD
Department of Gastroenterology, University of
Chicago, Chicago, Illinois

STEVEN H. DAYAN, MD
Department of Otolaryngology-Head and
Neck Surgery, Clinical Assistant Professor of
Otolaryngology, Chicago Center for Facial

Plastic Surgery; School of New Learning,
Adjunct Professor at DePaul University,
Chicago, Illinois

KARAN DHIR, MD
Assistant Clinical Professor, Department of
Head and Neck Surgery, University
of California-Harbor, Los Angeles,
Beverly Hills, California

JESSE KEVIN DUPLECHAIN, MD
Clinical Instructor, Department of
Otolaryngology, Tulane University Medical
School; The Aesthetic Center, Lafayette,
Louisiana

ANDREW A. JACONO, MD, FACS
Section Head, Facial Plastic and
Reconstructive Surgery, North Shore University
Hospital, Manhasset, New York; Clinical
Assistant Professor, Facial Plastic Surgery,
The New York Eye and Ear Infirmary, New York,
New York; Clinical Assistant Professor,
Department of Otorhinolaryngology-Head and
Neck Surgery, The Albert Einstein College of
Medicine, Bronx, New York; The New York
Center for Facial Plastic and Laser Surgery,
Great Neck, New York

MICHAEL E. JASIN, MD, FACS
Jasin Facial Rejuvenation Institute, Tampa, Florida

HEDYEH JAVIDNIA, MD
Division of Facial Plastic and Reconstructive Surgery, Department of Otolaryngology, UC Davis, Sacramento, California

JOHN JOSEPH, MD, FACS
Assistant Clinical Professor, Department of Head and Neck Surgery, University of California, Los Angeles

THEDA C. KONTIS, MD, FACS
Assistant Professor, Department of Otolaryngology-Head and Neck Surgery, Johns Hopkins Medical Institutions; Facial Plastic Surgicenter, LLC, Baltimore, Maryland

SAMUEL M. LAM, MD, FACS
Director, Willow Bend Wellness Center, Plano, Texas

MYRIAM LOYO, MD
Resident, Department of Otolaryngology–Head and Neck Surgery, Johns Hopkins Medical Institutions, Baltimore, Maryland

ALLISON T. PONTIUS, MD
Facial Plastic and Reconstructive Surgery, Williams' Center of Plastic Surgery Specialists, Latham, New York

JOSEPH J. ROUSSO, MD
The New York Center for Facial Plastic and Laser Surgery, Great Neck, New York

JONATHAN SYKES, MD, FACS
Division of Facial Plastic and Reconstructive Surgery, Department of Otolaryngology, UC Davis, Sacramento, California

ROBERT A. WEISS, MD, FAAD, FACPh
Associate Professor, Department of Dermatology, Johns Hopkins University School of Medicine; Director, The Maryland Laser, Skin, and Vein Institute, Hunt Valley, Baltimore, Maryland

EDWIN F. WILLIAMS III, MD, FACS
Director, Facial Plastic and Reconstructive Surgery, Williams' Center of Plastic Surgery Specialists, Latham, New York; Clinical Professor of Surgery, Division of Otolaryngology-Head and Neck Surgery, Department of Surgery, Albany Medical Center, Albany, New York

Contents

 The authors' procedure for the minimal-access deep-plane extended (MADE) facelift is presented in a video that accompanies this article

Because modern facelift patients desire a less-invasive approach or minimally invasive approach to reduce visible scarring and decrease the recovery phase, achieving the surgeon's goal of optimal, reliable, and long-term aesthetic results with few complications becomes a challenge. The authors use the terms minimal access and traditional access to describe rhytidectomy approaches based solely on incision size. A short-incision, minimal-access approach with a deep-plane extended dissection is presented. A preoperative physical examination maneuver to evaluate a patient's candidacy for a minimal-access approach and guidelines for when to include platysmaplasty with the procedure to further improve cervicomental contour are described.

This article describes the use of the endoscopic brow-lifting technique in addressing periorbital aging. This article discusses the advantages and disadvantage of the endoscopic versus traditional techniques of brow lifting and gives our treatment algorithm depending on patient needs.

 Dr Joseph demonstrates midface facial filling with Sculptra and discusses his preparation of the materials for tear trough and midface injection in a video that accompanies this article

Alloplastic facial implants and injectable fillers are currently used for facial rejuvenation and augmentation. Their respective roles in augmentation and volume replacement of the chin and midface are discussed. Treatment goals, patient selection, procedures, and patient recovery are detailed. In addition, there is a segment for surgeons presenting a decision algorithm for selecting surgical versus less-invasive or nonsurgical approaches for midface rejuvenation.

 Videos are provided of animation of combined deep fractional and superficial ablative treatments; resurfacing of the upper neck; and resurfacing of deep perioral rhytids accompanying this article

The author uses the pulsed ablative CO_2 laser regularly for skin rejuvenation. This decision is based on the gold standard status of the CO_2 modality and an innovative aftercare treatment shown in the author's practice to greatly reduce the complications of ablative pulsed CO_2 laser treatment. Depending on the patient and the severity of the skin condition, the author customizes each treatment, which may also include fractional CO_2 lasers, fat grafting, facelifting, or any combination of these techniques. This article presents a detailed description of the evolution of skin rejuvenation with lasers and the current role of lasers as an adjunct to face and necklift surgery.

 A video demonstrating injection of a patient with calcium hydroxylapatite in the midface and with hyaluronic acid in the tear trough can be viewed online

This article examines the increasing role of injectable fillers to treat midface aging and our approach to decision making regarding the use of fillers versus surgery. We discuss the volume changes of the aging midface and advocate taking an anatomic approach to correct these changes. We discuss our approach to patient selection and injection technique. Finally, we review potential complications from injectable fillers and discuss the management of complications.

With the advent of newer injectables with less immunogenicity and greater longevity, nonsurgical rhinoplasty has become a viable alternative to surgery. An understanding of the surgical anatomy of the nose, particularly in a postrhinoplasty patient, affords the physician injector the opportunity to better plan the injectable treatment. This article outlines the evolution of nonsurgical rhinoplasty and identifies properties to consider when selecting which dermal filler to use. It includes a description of the types of nasal deformities that can be treated with injectables, as well as the role of nonsurgical rhinoplasty in a comprehensive regimen for correction of nasal deformities.

Fat transfer is a cornerstone to managing facial aging and can represent a stand-alone procedure or be used in conjunction with other surgical treatments. Fat can also be used with fillers or as an alternative to fillers both for the benefit of educating surgeons and for improved patient communication to establish clear expectations of results. The surgeon should discuss these aspects with a patient in a preoperative setting to avoid false expectations. Fat is a bioactive substance and fat transfer should be avoided in very young patients, in those with weight instability, and in cases of asymmetric placement.

The aging neck is accompanied by an increase in submental fat, platysmal banding, and redundant dyspigmented skin. Creating a more acute cervicomental angle, distinct mandibular border, homogeneous skin tone, and smoother texture helps to achieve a more youthful appearance. The aesthetic provider's armamentarium has long had surgical techniques in the highest regard, but a new wave of minimally invasive procedures looks to offer a nonsurgical approach to cervicomental rejuvenation. Selecting the appropriate procedure for appropriate patients that will effectively meet their aesthetic goals and expectations is the core of successful neck rejuvenation.

Facial volume loss is an important component of facial aging and tends to present at an earlier age than other aspects of aging. Several surgical and nonsurgical products and techniques are available to replace volume loss associated with aging. One surgical technique uses a patient's fat cells to replace or augment volume deficiency. Poly-L–lactic acid (PLLA) injection is a nonsurgical option. This article compares these 2 volume augmentation procedures and discusses characteristics of facial aging, the consultation process involved in assessing individual volume loss, procedure details of autologous fat grafting and PLLA injection, the decision of PLLA versus autologous fat, and patient outcomes.

Botulinum toxin (BoNTA) has become the modern generation's treatment of choice for facial aging. Advanced uses of neurotoxin have treated specific areas of the face, in addition to the glabella, which is the only site for injection approved by the Food and Drug Administration. This article suggests that BoNTA has replaced surgical procedures that treat oral commissures, mild brow ptosis and brow asymmetries, and hypertrophic orbicularis oculi muscles. It is becoming increasingly used for lip asymmetry, platysmal banding, and necklift, although it has not replaced traditional procedures for the correction of these areas.

This article discusses autologous cell therapy for wrinkles in the face. Autologous fibroblast therapy is compared with dermal fillers. Study outcomes of LaViv are detailed, including a summary of adverse events. The technique for injection of autologous cells is described in addition to the duration of effect of treatment.

Advisory Board to Facial Plastic Surgery Clinics 2013

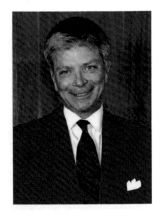
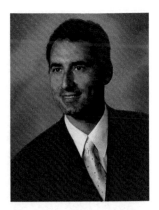
Facial Plastic Surgery Clinics is pleased to introduce the 2012-2013 **Advisory Board**.

Facial Plastic Surgery Clinics is widely available through the media of print, digital e-Reader, online via the Internet, and on iPad and smart phones.

Facial Plastic Surgery Clinics provides professionals access to pertinent point-of-care answers and current clinical information, along with comprehensive background information for deeper understanding.

Readers are welcome to contact the Clinics Editor or Board with comments.

BOARD MEMBERS 2013

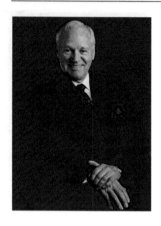

PETER A. ADAMSON, MD

Professor and Head
Division of Facial Plastic and Reconstructive Surgery
Department of Otolaryngology–Head and Neck Surgery
University of Toronto
Toronto, Ontario, Canada

Adamson Cosmetic Facial Surgery
Renaissance Plaza; 150 Bloor Street West; Suite M110
Toronto, Ontario M5S 2X9

416.323.3900
paa@dradamson.com
www.dradamson.com

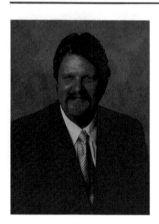

RICK DAVIS, MD

Voluntary Professor
The University of Miami Miller School of Medicine
Miami, Florida

The Center for Facial Restoration
1951 S.W. 172nd Ave; Suite 205
Miramar, Florida 33029

954.442.5191
drd@davisrhinoplasty.com
www.DavisRhinoplasty.com

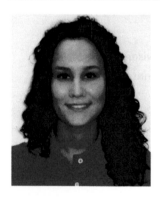

TATIANA DIXON, MD

University of Illinois at Chicago
Resident,
Department of Otolaryngology–Head and Neck Surgery

1855 W. Taylor
Chicago, IL 60612

312.996.6555
TFeuer1@UIC.EDU

STEVEN FAGIEN, MD, FACS

Aesthetic Eyelid Plastic Surgery
660 Glades Road; Suite 210
Boca Raton, Florida 33431

561.393.9898
sfagien@aol.com

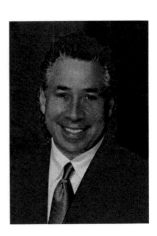

GREG KELLER, MD

Clinical Professor of Surgery, Head and Neck,
David Geffen School of Medicine,
University of California, Los Angeles;

Keller Facial Plastic Surgery
221 W. Pueblo St. Ste A
Santa Barbara, CA 93105

805.687.6408
faclft@aol.com
www.gregorykeller.com

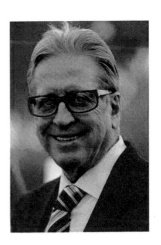

THEDA C. KONTIS, MD

Assistant Professor, Johns Hopkins Hospital
Facial Plastic Surgicenter, Ltd.
1838 Greene Tree Road, Suite 370
Baltimore, MD 21208

410.486.3400
tckontis@aol.com
www.facialplasticsurgerymd.com
www.facial-plasticsurgery.com

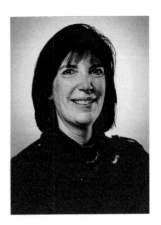

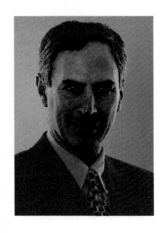

IRA D. PAPEL, MD

Facial Plastic Surgicenter
Associate Professor
The Johns Hopkins University
1838 Greene Tree Road, Suite 370
Baltimore, MD 21208

410.486.3400
idpmd@aol.com
www.facial-plasticsurgery.com

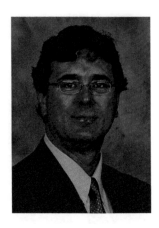

SHERARD A. TATUM, MD

Professor of Otolaryngology and
Pediatrics Cleft and Craniofacial Center
Division of Facial Plastic Surgery
Upstate Medical University
750 E. Adams St.
Syracuse, NY 13210

315.464.4636
TatumS@upstate.edu
www.upstate.edu

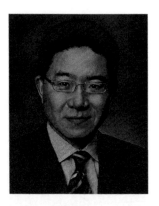

TOM D. WANG, MD

Professor
Facial Plastic and Reconstructive Surgery
Oregon Health & Science University
3181 Southwest Sam Jackson Park Road
Portland, OR 97239

503.494.5678
wangt@ohsu.edu
www.ohsu.edu/drtomwang

FACIAL PLASTIC SURGERY CLINICS OF NORTH AMERICA

FORTHCOMING ISSUES

Hair Restoration
Raymond Konior, MD and Stephen Gabel, MD, *Editors*

Complications in Facial Plastic Surgery
Richard L. Goode, MD and Samuel P. Most, MD, *Editors*

Techniques in Facial Plastic Surgery: Discussion and Debate, Volume 2
Fred Fedok, MD and Robert Kellman, MD, *Editors*

RECENT ISSUES

February 2013
Facial Skin: Contemporary Topics for the Surgeon
David B. Hom, MD, FACS and
Adam Ingraffea, MD, FAAD, FACMS, *Editors*

November 2012
Nonmelanoma Skin Cancer of the Head and Neck
Cemal Cingi, *Editor*

August 2012
Techniques in Facial Plastic Surgery: Discussion and Debate
Fred G. Fedok, MD and Robert M. Kellman, MD, *Editors*

RELATED INTEREST

Clinics in Plastic Surgery January 2013 (Vol. 40, Issue 1)
Brow and Upper Eyelid Surgery: Multispecialty Approach
Babak Azizzadeh and Guy Massry, *Editors*

Preface
Minimal Facial Plastic Surgery Procedures ... Maximal Results?

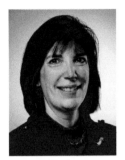

Theda C. Kontis, MD, FACS
Editor

This year marks the 20th Anniversary of *Facial Plastic Surgery Clinics*. I know this because on my bookshelf rests every edition since the flagship issue on Open Rhinoplasty published in August 1993. The first issue on Minimally Invasive Procedures was published in 2001 and discussed chemical peels, lasers, and endoscopic approaches to facial surgery. Botulinum toxin for facial aesthetics was FDA approved in 2002 and, only 1 year later, an entire issue of *Facial Plastic Surgery Clinics* was dedicated to the cosmetic use of Botox. Now, in 2013, we are asking if more invasive procedures are becoming or have become obsolete with the advent of newer, less invasive procedures.

We all agree that the practice of medicine evolves. Older physicians are likely not practicing the way they did 20 years ago. As our knowledge of facial aging improves in addition to the development of new materials, instruments, and techniques, we are able to improve our treatment outcomes with increased safety, less scarring, and faster recoveries. Medicine benefits from the advances in technology, which become both smaller and less expensive over time. We respond to the desires of our patients, who want less invasive procedures with minimal recovery. But are we still able to provide maximal results with minimal procedures?

For several years now, I have been thinking about how we are now able to perform many cosmetic procedures without resorting to more aggressive techniques of the past. I don't perform coronal brow lifts, oral commissure-plasties, or vermillion advancements anymore. I learned how to augment the face with fat and fillers and how to sculpt the face with neurotoxins. I have abandoned ablative laser resurfacing of the face for gentler fractional resurfacing. I was excited to be given the task of posing directed questions to leaders in our field to ask them their thoughts about this less invasive trend in cosmetic procedures. I am grateful to the contributors to this issue and I appreciate the thought that each of the authors placed on their assigned topic. I applaud their insight into the difficult questions posed to them.

I am certain the reader will enjoy reading how far we have advanced in the last 20 years and how technological advancements have continued to shape our field. It will be interesting to watch how the titles of *Facial Plastic Surgery Clinics* will trend over the *next* 20 years. I suspect not only will the materials improve and techniques become noninvasive but also the "books" on my bookshelf will be replaced by the newest and most compact forms of electronic media!

Theda C. Kontis, MD, FACS
Johns Hopkins Hospital
Facial Plastic Surgicenter, Ltd
1838 Greene Tree Road, Suite 370
Baltimore, MD 21208, USA

E-mail address:
tckontis@aol.com

Facial Plast Surg Clin N Am 21 (2013) xv
http://dx.doi.org/10.1016/j.fsc.2013.02.011
1064-7406/13/$ – see front matter © 2013 Published by Elsevier Inc.

facialplastic.theclinics.com

The Modern Minimally Invasive Face Lift
Has It Replaced the Traditional Access Approach?

Andrew A. Jacono, MD[a,b,c,d,*], Joseph J. Rousso, MD[d]

KEYWORDS

- Facelift • Minimally invasive facelift • Rhytidectomy • SMAS • Deep plane facelift • Vertical facelift
- Short scar facelift • Minimal access facelift • Facial rejuvenation • Modern facelift • MADE facelift

KEY POINTS

- Current trends in surgery are evolving towards less invasive techniques.
- Minimal access techniques should provide long-term aesthetic results with few complications.
- A short incision, minimal access approach with a deep plane extended dissection is described and guidelines for its use are discussed in detail.

 The authors' procedure for the minimal-access deep-plane extended (MADE) facelift is presented in a video that accompanies this article at http://www.facialplastic.theclinics.com/

INTRODUCTION

With the increasing popularity and societal acceptance of cosmetic surgery over the last 3 decades, several novel rhytidectomy techniques have emerged. Current trends in surgery are evolving toward less invasive techniques. Therefore, it is no surprise that subspecialties of minimally invasive surgery have evolved and patients actively seek surgeons trained in these methods. The authors think that, in rhytidectomy surgery, the term *minimally invasive* translates into patients' desire for

1. A smaller incision and, therefore, less scarring
2. A shorter postoperative recovery
3. Less risk

The result of this mindset is that patients are shying away from longer incision techniques. These techniques include approaches that enter into the temporal scalp with consequential hair loss and long posterior auricular/occipital scalp incisions that prevent patients from wearing their hair up in a ponytail. Some of the more recently popularized modifications promote the use of a vertical vector of lift, which limits the need for posterior auricular/occipital incisions and scars, such as that seen in the minimal-access cranial suspension (MACS) lift.[1] Although the authors do not use the MACS lift, they incorporate the principal of lifting both the Superficial Musculo-Aponeurotic System (SMAS) and superficial tissues in a more vertical vector in their technique that is described in this article.

Misconceptions of Lunchtime Lifts

This patient mindset has also led to the popularization of terms, such as *lunchtime facelifts*, that lead the consumer to think that a procedure and

[a] Facial Plastic and Reconstructive Surgery, North Shore University Hospital, Manhasset, NY, USA; [b] Facial Plastic Surgery, The New York Eye and Ear Infirmary, New York, NY, USA; [c] Department of Otorhinolaryngology, Head and Neck Surgery, The Albert Einstein College of Medicine, Bronx, NY, USA; [d] The New York Center for Facial Plastic and Laser Surgery, 440 Northern Boulevard, Great Neck, NY 11021, USA
* Corresponding author. 440 Northern Boulevard, Great Neck, NY 11021.
E-mail address: drjacono@gmail.com

Facial Plast Surg Clin N Am 21 (2013) 171–189
http://dx.doi.org/10.1016/j.fsc.2013.02.002
1064-7406/13/$ – see front matter © 2013 Elsevier Inc. All rights reserved.

recovery can occur over 1 hour. Full chains of surgical centers offer these procedures promoting a minimal recovery time. Unfortunately, there are several misconceptions that arise with buzzword marketing, and this may lead to patient dissatisfaction. Although less invasive procedures may have some component of decreased recovery time, the lunchtime facelift tends to understate the true extent of postoperative edema, ecchymosis, and overall recovery that is encountered. Even in a short skin-flap SMAS plication rhytidectomy, early recovery, including bruising and swelling, can extend for 1 to 2 weeks, which is hardly lunchtime.

The misconception is further compounded by the fact that, although patients want a minimal procedure, they do not want a minimal or subtle result or a result that lasts a minimal or short duration. Most patients expect results of a facelift to address the face, including the jawline (jowls) and drooping cheeks and neck. Also, they expect it to last 5 to 10 years. Patients anticipate the efficacy of a minimally invasive technique to be comparable with a more invasive technique. Although a surgeon can manage expectations and describe that a procedure will have a partial correction in certain areas or will have less longevity, it is the authors' experience that patients are dissatisfied when they have residual facial ptosis, jowling, and neck redundancy.

Surgeons' View of Minimally Invasive Facelifts

To most surgeons, a minimally invasive facelift is synonymous with a limited incision, short skin-flap elevation, and an SMAS plication or imbrication. The senior author (A.A.J.) has essentially abandoned this technique because the authors have experienced a high recurrence of facial ptosis over a 1- to 2-year period. A recent review of the plastic surgery literature has demonstrated a lack of consensus about whether more manipulation of the SMAS and deep facial tissues improves outcomes in rhytidectomy.[2] There are a few studies suggesting no difference in outcomes at 1 year when comparing minimal SMAS manipulation techniques with more significant manipulation, but these studies only used subjective photographic analysis by physicians.[3,4] They did not account for patient satisfaction with the procedure, and the cohorts had small treatment groups with only 20 patients. A study focusing on patient dissatisfaction after rhytidectomy caused by the recurrence of facial ptosis demonstrated that either the SMAS plication technique used in the MACS lift or the SMASectomy approach have a dissatisfaction rate requiring a tuck-up procedure in 50% of cases at 2 years.[5] Others have demonstrated a 21.7% dissatisfaction rate at 1 year caused by

persistent jowling after a short skin-flap SMAS plication facelift, which necessitated a tuck-up procedure.[6] This finding is not surprising because the short-term efficacy of SMAS plication was noted by Aufrecht and Baker,[7] who first described plicating the SMAS in the 1960s. Other studies demonstrated no benefit when plicating the SMAS versus a skin-only rhytidectomy at 1 year.[8,9]

After Hamra's[10] description of the deep-plane rhytidectomy, Kamer and Frankel[11] demonstrated a 97% patient satisfaction rate in a cohort of 335 patients undergoing the deep-plane technique, decreasing the tuck-up rate at 1 year to 3.3% when compared with a 11.4% tuck-up rate with an extended SMAS flap cohort of 279 patients. The greater longevity of rhytidectomy techniques that elevate an extended SMAS flap was also shown in another study whereby the average length of time from the primary to secondary facelift in patients repeating their rhytidectomy was 11.9 years.[12]

MADE Lift

Because of the senior author's (A.A.J.) experience, and supported by the aforementioned data, he has evolved to a rhytidectomy procedure that incorporates a shorter incision with an extended deep-plane dissection that has been described as a MADE facelift or minimal-access deep-plane extended vertical vector facelift.[13] This technique is the subject of this article. The authors' tuck-up rate on 153 patients at 1 year of 3.9% was published in its original description and has been consistent at 3.0% after the 1-year follow-up of 254 patients. The shorter incision is possible by incorporating a more vertical vector of skin excision as originally described in the MACS lift.

The MADE lift includes a more extensive dissection of the cheek, including the release of the zygomatic osseocutaneous ligaments with vertical elevation of the malar fat pad for midface improvement. This vertical elevation is not possible without the release of the zygomatico-cutaneous ligaments and more extensive midface dissection. It has been recently shown that the zygomatic ligament is the strongest of the facial retaining ligaments and has limited elasticity.[14] This finding suggests that without the release of this region, superficial suturing techniques will have little effect on midface improvement. This release and vertical elevation creates a superior stacking of the malar fat pad, which adds volume to the cheek and recreates the heart-shape face of youth.

Recovery Time with the MADE Lift

The questions is whether this shorter-incision deep-plane approach, although potentially more efficacious, is commensurate with the patients' desire for minimal surgery because it may create a longer recovery. Interestingly, it has been the authors' experience that a deep-plane rhytidectomy, which involves the elevation of the skin and SMAS as a composite flap without delaminating them, is associated with a shorter recovery than when they performed a skin flap in rhytidectomy with a separate SMAS tightening. The authors think this decreased bruising is caused by the avascular nature of the deep-plane flap fascial dissection when compared with the highly vascular plane of dissection within the subdermal plexus during skin-flap elevation in traditional rhytidectomy. When a skin flap is elevated, any bruising is also more superficial and, therefore, more visible during recovery when compared with deep-plane dissection. The authors also have noticed more rapid resolution of bruising and faster healing of incision lines. The authors think that this is caused by the greater blood supply of the deep-plane flap. Deep-plane surgery preserves the transverse facial artery, which acts as an axial blood supply to the facelift lift flap, while this vessel is disconnected from the skin during skin flap elevation in standard rhytidectomy.[15]

Edema and Lymphatic Drainage in Facelift

It is often suggested that either deep-plane dissection or elevation of an SMAS flap is associated with greater postoperative edema, but a recent study does not support this conclusion. Lymphoscintigraphy during the postoperative period shows that the depth of dissection disrupts lymphatic drainage of the face the same as simple skin-flap elevation.[16] It is the length of flap elevation and not its depth that determines its effects on lymphatic drainage of the face. In fact, this study demonstrated that all approaches studied, which included a skin flap with SMAS plication and composite rhytidectomy, have a subtotal recovery of lymphatic pathways within 3 months and complete return-to-baseline drainage pattern after 6 months, regardless of the surgical technique. This finding also explains why patients typically like their results more at 3 months when their face has increased volumization as a result of some residual postoperative edema than after 6 months to a year when all edema has resolved.

Risks Involved in Facelift

Patients looking for a minimally invasive procedure often desire a procedure with less risk. All rhytidectomy approaches have 3 possible major complications:

1. Hematoma
2. Skin slough
3. Facial nerve paresis

The incidence of hematoma is usually quoted between 1.8% and 9%, but higher or lower hematoma rates have not been identified in any particular approach.[17,18]

The rate of skin slough in rhytidectomy is greater in techniques that require a long skin flap to be elevated because the main blood supply to the skin flap is random based on the subdermal plexus; the longer the flap, the greater the risk of necrosis. Because of this, shorter skin flaps do have a lower rate of necrosis. Although deep-plane flaps are longer flaps, they maintain a thicker flap with the preservation of the transverse facial artery as noted and, thus, have a theoretical lower rate of skin necrosis. This feature makes a long deep-plane flap more favorable than a long skin flap. The senior author has demonstrated a 0% skin slough rate in patients actively smoking during the preoperative and postoperative phase when undergoing deep-plane rhytidectomy.[19] This finding supports the idea that the greater blood supply of the deep-plane flap reduces the risk of necrosis.

Facial nerve paresis is a concern for both the patients and surgeon. Although staying superficial to the nerves by performing plication of the SMAS implies less risk, facial nerves can be lassoed with suturing techniques creating nerve injury.[20] Further, there have not been any studies showing increased rates of temporary or permanent facial nerve paresis related to more aggressive lifting of the SMAS in SMAS flap or deep-plane rhytidectomy with a careful and experienced technique. In fact, a series of 2500 consecutive deep-plane facelifts had no permanent facial nerve injury.[21] The authors have reported a temporary facial nerve neuropraxia rate of 1.3% and no permanent facial nerve injuries,[13] which is within the reported incidence of 2.1% temporary neuropraxia reported in a survey of more than 12 000 facelifts.[22]

Surgical Approach Options

Because the MADE procedure results in a shorter incision, addresses the midface, jawline and neck, has a more rapid healing phase, and has a low rate of complications, it is the procedure the authors offer for their patients seeking a minimally invasive procedure. The authors offer primary surgical patients 2 approaches: a *minimal-access* (short incision) deep-plane vertical facelift (MADE) or a *traditional-access* (longer incision) deep-plane facelift. The key to the MADE approach's shorter incision (not requiring a posterior auricular/occipital scalp limb) is the vertical vector of the lift. It is also less invasive because it does not require a separate midline platysmal tightening procedure because the deep plane is extended below the mandible and creates a widely undermined lateral platysmal flap, which corrects midline platysmal redundancy. This lack of a midline platysmoplasty makes the procedure duration shorter by obviating an additional platysmaplasty. It can be used in most aging face candidates with mild to moderate rhytidosis facialis, usually in the 40s to the 60s.

Poor candidates for this approach include those with more severe facial ptosis and poor anatomy, including retrognathia, low anterior hyoid, and severe platysmal redundancy. They require a traditional-access deep-plane facelift often combined with a midline platysmaplasty. The authors' traditional-access approach incorporates a longer postauricular incision that extends into the occipital scalp and a submental incision for anterior platysmal plication.

The authors not only describe their short-incision, extended deep-plane, vertical vector facelift surgical technique but also a method to evaluate patients' candidacy for a minimal-access approach based on a preoperative physical examination maneuver. The authors also provide guidelines to help the surgeon decide when to include Platysmaplasty with the procedure to further improve the cervicomental contour. The authors' experience with 342 patients with this approach is presented.

Preoperative Evaluation and Candidacy

The authors have developed a basic decision algorithm for determining whether patients are candidates for minimal access or traditional access to a facelift. The preoperative physical examination of patients is the most decisive factor in the determination of candidacy for a short-incision deep-plane rhytidectomy. This examination includes observing how the face and neck redrapes when traction is placed on the skin along the vertical vectors of this facelift technique. The authors have had success with patients aged from 40 to 70 years, even if there is significant anterior platysmal cording and submental skin excess. Anatomic variants that may predispose to failures in the submental region with this technique include those with retrognathia, low anterior hyoid, and a short vertical height of the neck. In these cases, more aggressive submental surgery is required. The additional procedures that address unfavorable cervicomental contour issues include submental liposuction, platysmal plication, subplatysmal fat excision, and/or anterior digastric plication.

A physical examination technique that the authors use to determine candidacy for the MADE vertical facelift involves traction on the facial skin to evaluate the vertical and horizontal components of the neck; the authors call this the facial redraping capacity (**Fig. 1**). This technique helps determine whether patients are candidates for sparing the posterior hairline incision of traditional facelifts. The deep-plane entry point is a line that courses from the angle of the mandible to the lateral canthus.

- The surgeon places 3 fingers at the deep-plane entry point on both sides of the face and moves the skin vertically to assess whether the submental and platysmal skin laxity is corrected.
- If the submental area is corrected, then there is no posterior hairline limb incision or any anterior platysmal surgery necessary.
- If patients still have significant horizontal neck skin excess with this maneuver, and platysmal cording exists, then an abbreviated incision is not advisable. The neck redundancy will exist and recur postoperatively. A posterior auricular hairline incision to remove the horizontal neck laxity and anterior platysma plication for midline platysmal redundancy would then be necessary.

Another guideline used when deciding whether to add a platysmaplasty to the facelift procedure or not is based on anatomic studies. Extending a traditional deep-plane rhytidectomy inferiorly to release the lateral platysma and cervical retaining ligaments of the platysma to the sternocleidomastoid muscle achieves greater lateral motion of the midline platysma, in fact 554% more than using lateral platysmal plication suturing.[23] In this study, the average redraping of the midline platysma was 2.4 cm. Because of this, the authors are more likely to perform a midline platysmaplasty to resect excess medial platysma and plicate the two sides in the midline when the platysmal divergence approaches 3 cm.

OPERATIVE TECHNIQUE

See the Video on the MADE facelift procedure online at http://www.facialplastic.theclinics.com/.

Preoperative Marking

- With patients sitting upright, several important anatomic landmarks are outlined

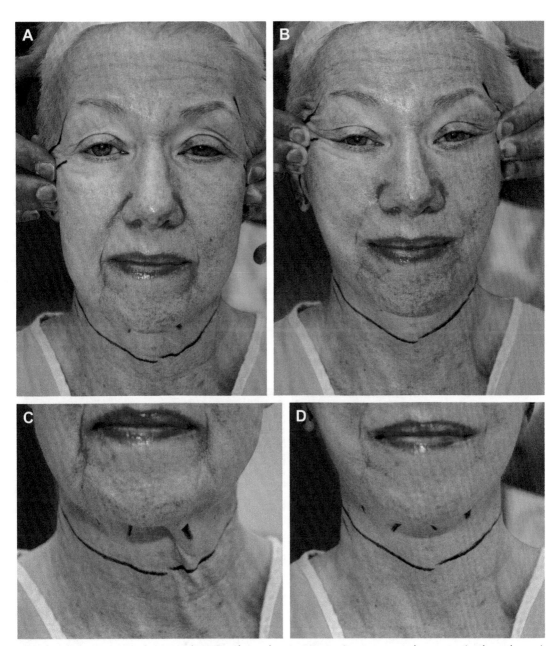

Fig. 1. (*A, B*) The patient is shown undergoing the authors' preoperative maneuver demonstrating how the anticipated vertical vector elevation along a deep-plane entry point in the face will treat platysmal cording and submental laxity. For this part of the examination, the surgeon places 3 fingers at the deep-plane entry point (the line coursing from the angle of the mandible to the lateral canthus) on both sides of the face and moves the skin vertically to assess whether the submental and platysmal skin laxity is corrected with this tension. (*C, D*) Close-up views of the submental region with preoperative maneuver. If the submental area is corrected, no posterior hairline limb incision or any anterior platysmal surgery is necessary. If patients still have significant horizontal neck skin excess with this maneuver and platysmal cording still exists, the abbreviated incision associated with the authors' MADE lift is not advisable because neck redundancy will persist or recur postoperatively.

preoperatively, including the path of the temporal branch of the facial nerve and the deep-plane entry point, which proceeds from the angle of the mandible to the lateral canthus.

- The anterior temporal hairline is marked beginning 1.5 cm above the tail of the eyebrow and tracked along the inferior hairline of the sideburn, into the hairless recess between sideburn and auricle, turning downward into the preauricular crease, continuing post-tragally, and then following the crease of the lobule-facial junction.

- The mark is carried behind the earlobe-facial junction, superiorly onto the posterior concha for 2 cm (**Fig. 2**).

Surgical procedure

Anesthesia The MADE vertical facelift can be performed under local anesthesia, conscious sedation, or general anesthesia. In the last 2 years, approximately 40% of the authors' patients elected to undergo this procedure under local anesthesia (0.5% lidocaine with 1:200 000 units of epinephrine, mixed in equal parts with 0.25% bupivacaine with 1:200 000 units of epinephrine); the remaining patients chose intravenous sedation. The local anesthetic is infiltrated along the incision and over the area of subcutaneous and deep-plane dissection.

Incision and undermining
Incision

- The skin incision is made with a No. 10 blade.

Surgical tips: *If the MADE vertical facelift is being performed as a sole procedure, the temporal hair tuft sparing incision was extended superiorly to a greater degree than in a more traditional facelift because of the vertical vector of skin redraping. Because the majority of the redundant ptotic skin is removed in the temporal region, there is no need to extend the incision in the posterior auricular/occipital scalp. More horizontal vectors of skin excision require the posterior limb because the extra skin is shifted behind the ear. Not lengthening the incision in the posterior auricular/occipital scalp in a more horizontally redraping of the skin in a facelift would create postauricular deformities and lumpiness from skin that is bunched up and not removed. If the facelift is taking place concurrently with a lateral temporal lift, the anterior temporal hairline incision is shortened.*

- The temporal hairline incisions are MADE in a trichophytic fashion perpendicular to the hair shafts to allow hair regrowth through the scar once the facelift flap was trimmed and inset.

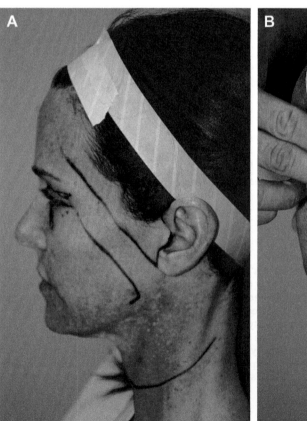
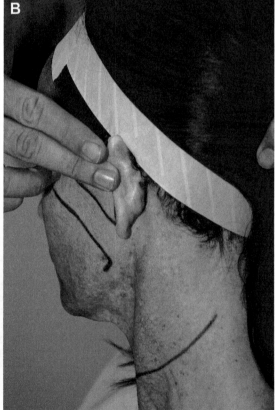

Fig. 2. (*A*) Preauricular and (*B*) postauricular rhytidectomy incision markings. Notice the posterior auricular incision limited to the skin of the conchal bowl. Also note the temporal hair tuft sparing excision with extensions superiorly to allow for vertical skin elevation.

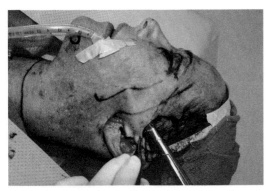

Fig. 3. The skin is elevated in a subcutaneous plane to the level of the deep-plane entry point.

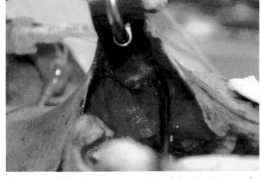

Fig. 5. Facelift scissors are used to bluntly elevate the sub-SMAS plane in the inferior cheek portion of the deep-plane flap.

- The earlobe is held in a retracted position for counter-tension.
- The incision is extended 2 cm superior to the earlobe-facial junction along the posterior concha of the ear, never crossing onto the mastoid skin. This maneuver conceals the incision even when patients wear their hair in a ponytail postoperatively.

Dissection
- The subcutaneous flap is initially dissected with a No. 10 scalpel and Brown forceps.
- The dissection is continued with facelift scissors, with the tines pointing upward.
- The surgeon consistently palpates the thickness of the flap for any irregularities with the nondominant hand.
- The subcutaneous dissection is then continued anteriorly to the deep-plane entry point, a line drawn from the angle of the mandible to the lateral canthus, and inferiorly 5 cm below the hyoid bone (**Fig. 3**).

- An incision is then MADE through the SMAS with a No. 10 scalpel, extending from the angle of the mandible to the lateral canthus (the deep-plane entry point) (**Fig. 4**).
- From that point, the subcutaneous flap and SMAS are dissected bluntly as one compound unit anteriorly in a sub-SMAS plane in the inferior cheek.
- Facelift scissors are then inserted and spread perpendicular to the branches of the facial nerve (**Fig. 5**).
- The plane of dissection is then advanced with a blunt dissector (model 502–5Z; Karl Storz, Tuttlingen, Germany) anteriorly to the level of the facial artery and inferiorly to 4 cm below the angle of the mandible.

Surgical tips: The zygomatico-cutaneous ligaments were initially left intact in the midface, and blunt dissection with a facelift scissors is used to identify the supraorbicularis oculi plane. Once this plane is identified, blunt finger dissection of

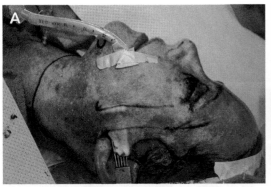
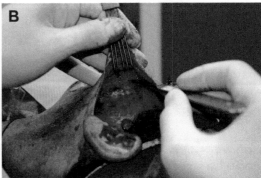

Fig. 4. (*A*) A pointed rake retractor is used to engage the tissues at the deep-plane entry point for counter-traction. (*B*) The deep plane is entered sharply with a No. 10 blade from the angle of the mandible to the lateral canthus while applying vertical tension with the retractor.

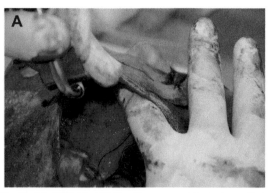

Fig. 6. (*A*) After identifying the supraorbicularis oculi plane, blunt finger dissection can be performed. (*B*) Finger-assisted malar elevation is continued over the midface superior to the zygomatico-cutaneous ligaments.

the midface tissues superior to these ligaments is easily performed and continues superficial to the zygomaticus major muscle (**Fig. 6**).

- This superior dissection plane continues medially ending at the nasolabial fold.
- In between the inferior cheek SMAS dissection and the superior dissection of the midface are the zygomatico-cutaneous ligaments that limit motion of the midface. At that point, they are divided sharply with a No. 10 blade and the dissection plane is continued bluntly with vertical spreading via facelift scissors, remaining in a plane superficial to the zygomaticus major musculature, thus connecting the superior and inferior pockets (**Fig. 7**).

Surgical tips: After the ligaments are released, this dissection yields a thick musculocutaneous flap comprised of skin and the malar fat pad of the

cheek superiorly and the SMAS and platysma inferiorly, which extends to the nasolabial fold (**Fig. 8**). This process releases the malar mound, including the malar fat pad, and allows the midface to be elevated vertically.

- Attention is then turned to the dissection of the deep-plane flap at the angle of the mandible.

Surgical tips: In the deep-plane facelift described by Hamra,[10] the deep plane is not dissected below the angle of the mandible, and the platysma is plicated to the mastoid region superficially in the preplatysmal plane. In this procedure, the SMAS, platysma, and anterior border of the sternocleidomastoid muscle interface are dissected, extending the deep plane below the angle of the mandible into the neck for 5 to 6 cm.

- An intraoperative marking is MADE from the deep-plane entry point at the angle of the mandible and extends inferiorly along the fascial attachments of the anterior border of

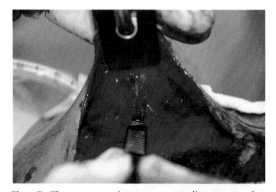

Fig. 7. The zygomatico-cutaneous ligaments that separate the superior and inferior deep-plane dissections are connected using sharp dissection with a No. 10 blade that continues on top of the zygomaticus major. This procedure can also be accomplished with blunt scissor dissection.

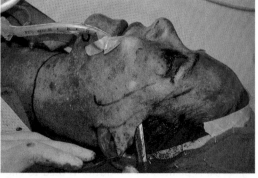

Fig. 8. Deep-plane flap elevated to the nasolabial fold with complete release of midface and cheek.

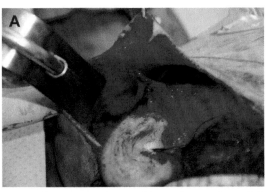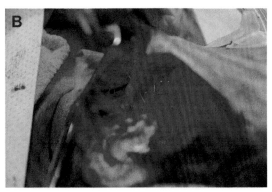

Fig. 9. (*A*) Intraoperative markings of extension of the deep-plane entry point 5 cm below the angle of the mandible to create an extended lateral platysmal flap. The platysma is released from its dense cervical attachments to the sternocleidomastoid muscle. (*B*) Platysmal flap after blunt dissection.

the sternocleidomastoid muscle to the platysma.

- The fascial attachments are released with a No. 15 scalpel while the assistant holds the edges of the tissue with Adson-Brown forceps.
- The dissection is continued under the platysma, 5 to 6 cm below the angle of the mandible.
- This important maneuver releases the dense fascial attachments of the platysma from the sternocleidomastoid muscle, which allows for greater mobilization (**Fig. 9**).
- The last step before vertical suspension of the deep-plane flap and extended lateral platysmal flap is dissection of a cuff along the deep-plane entry point. This cuff creates a tongue of tissue to facilitate suture suspension of the flap. The cuff is created with small snips of facelift scissors.
- Intraoperatively, hemostasis is achieved with bipolar cautery, and the tissues are irrigated with gentamycin irrigant. A No. 10 French Blake drain with a Jackson-Pratt bulb is placed into the patients' upper neck, with the puncture site behind the ear.

Suspension sutures

- A total of three 3-0 nylon suspension sutures are placed with a PS-2 needle to suspend the flap to the temporalis fascia such that the flap was advanced with a vertical vector with great tension on the SMAS but none on the skin.

Surgical tips: *The vector for ideal flap repositioning is determined by rotating directly horizontal (0°) and moved toward the vertical axis (90°). As the flap is moved, careful attention is given to the submental area, jawline, and midface. The*

angle that results in the greatest reduction of submental laxity and jowling, without flattening the midface (as seen with overly horizontal flap redraping) or creating malar bunching and lateral-facial pleats (as seen with overly vertical flap redraping), is used.

- Firm bites 1.0 to 1.5 cm long and 0.5 cm deep are placed into the cuff of the SMAS (dissected earlier in the procedure) in a horizontal mattress fashion. These 3 sutures are run from the leading edge of the composite flap at the deep-plane entry point to the deep temporal fascia (**Fig. 10**).

Surgical tips: *This vertical redraping of the face above the mandible reduces vertical platysmal redundancy but limits the available platysma for superolateral redraping. Therefore, after vertical suspension, a lateral platysmal myotomy of the extended subplatysmal flap of 3 to 4 cm is performed approximately 1 cm below the mandibular*

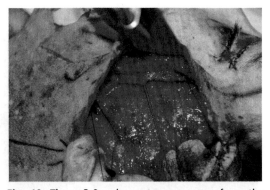

Fig. 10. Three 3-0 nylon sutures are run from the leading edge of the composite flap at the deep-plane entry point to the deep temporal fascia in a vertical vector.

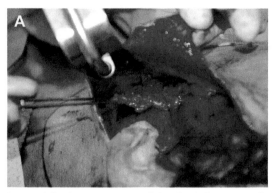
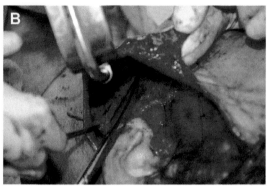

Fig. 11. (*A*) After suspension of the cheek flap vertically, the lateral platysmal flap is under vertical tension. (*B*) A lateral platysmal myotomy is performed 1 cm below the angle of the mandible to allow for superolateral positioning and tightening of the platysmal to the mastoid fascia.

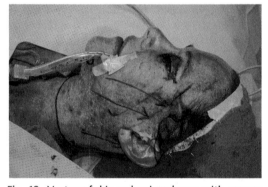

Fig. 12. Vector of skin redraping shown with arrows. Notice the region of most of the skin excision is in the pretemporal area and not the postauricular region, thus limiting the need for an extended occipital hairline incision.

angle (**Fig. 11**). *This practice allows for the separation of the vertical vector in the face from the superolateral vector on the platysma, which is required for durable neck rejuvenation.*

- A fourth suspension suture is placed along the extended lateral platysmal flap. This suture is anchored to the mastoid fascia and pulled in a superolateral vector. If we think of the vertical vector as representing an inverted bucket handle, the vertical suspension supports the submental region.

Skin redraping and resection Similar to the MACS lift, one of the most important features of the MADE vertical lift is vertical skin redraping. The traditional deep-plane facelift has a superolateral component of skin redraping in the face, causing skin excess in the postauricular and earlobe areas, which necessitates a posterior hairline limb incision for redraping. Alternatively, the skin redraping in a more vertical technique places most of the excess skin anteriorly, with minimal skin excision required posterior to the lobule (**Fig. 12**). Note

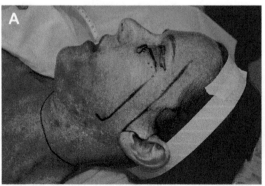
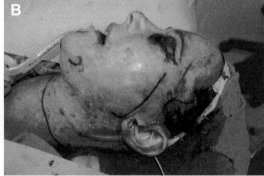

Fig. 13. Preoperative (*A*) and postoperative (*B*) views highlighting the volume of tissue motion as evidenced by the lateral and superior motion of the deep-plane entry point.

that the skin excision follows the suspension of the deep plane because the SMAS and skin are not delaminated in this composite technique. Excising skin vertically on both sides has a tightening effect on the skin in the submental region. The authors routinely find that the deep-plane entry point essentially merges with the newly created incision line (**Fig. 13**).

- Intraoperatively, the skin excision of the cheek flap is performed by following the anterior temporal hairline.
- Subcutaneous, buried, 4-0 vicryl sutures are placed in the anterior temporal hairline to minimize the spreading of the temporal incision and minimize any scarring.

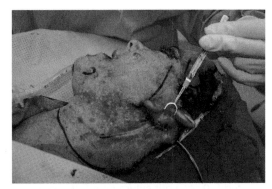

Fig. 14. Postauricular sutured incision line at completion of rhytidectomy. Note posterior auricular incision limited to the concha.

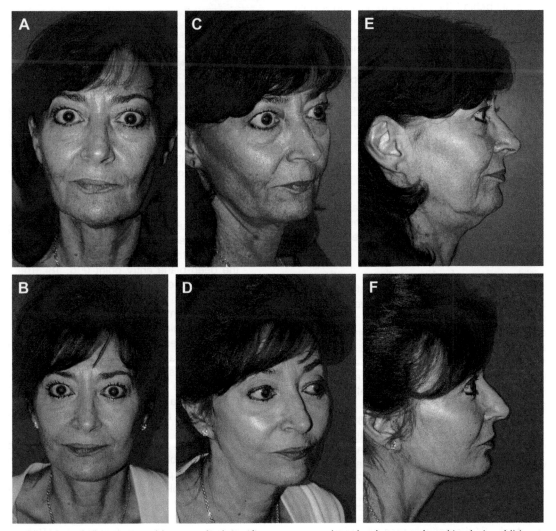

Fig. 15. (*A, C, E*) This 56-year-old woman had significant concerns about her heavy neck and jowls, in addition to midfacial ptosis and infraorbital hollowing. (*B, D, F*) Twelve months after MADE rhytidectomy, lower lid blepharoplasty with fat transposition. Note the youthful cervicomental region and rejuvenated infraorbital-malar contour. The vector of lift for this patient was 60°.

- The skin is everted with vertical mattress sutures.
- Sometimes the temporal incision must be continued superiorly for another 1 to 3 cm to remove the excess skin in patients with more advanced aging and rhytidosis; this avoids bunching of the skin in the superior portion of the anterior temporal hairline incision.
- The anterior facial incisions is closed with a 5-0 nylon suture on a P-3 needle, and the post-tragal incision is closed with an interrupted 5-0 plain gut suture on a P-3 needle.
- The earlobe is pulled upward and has to be set back with a small skin incision to place it back in its natural position.
- The posterior neck skin is pulled up vertically behind the earlobe to support it postoperatively, preventing a pixie ear deformity and elongation of the earlobe. Again, this does not require a posterior limb hairline incision.
- A 4-0 vicryl suture is used to support the neck skin flap in the retroauricular region immediately behind the concha to prevent any traction or distortion of the ear lobe.
- The postauricular incisions are closed with a 4-0 nylon suture (**Fig. 14**).

Surgical outcomes and results

The authors have performed 323 consecutive facelifts over a 33-month period (March 2009 to November 2011); each case was considered for a short-incision approach with a 1-year follow-up (**Figs. 15** and **16**).

Initial series of 181 patients undergoing a facelift In the authors' first series of 181 consecutive facelift patients,[13] 28 (15.5%) were not candidates for the MADE vertical lift because of anatomic variants, including retrognathia, a low anterior hyoid, short vertical height of the neck, and excessive platysmal laxity and cording (**Fig. 17**). This 15.5% required a posterior auricular incision extending into the occipital hairline and a submentoplasty.

The remaining 153 patients (84.5% of the total caseload) underwent a facelift with the MADE technique. The average age of these patients was 57.8 years (range, 36–75 years), and the average length of follow-up was 12.7 months.

- Six patients (3.9%) from the authors' series underwent a revision at 1 year postoperatively. Of the patients presenting for revision surgery, 3 patients required a tuck-up procedure, 2 patients required direct excision of submental neck skin, and 1 patient

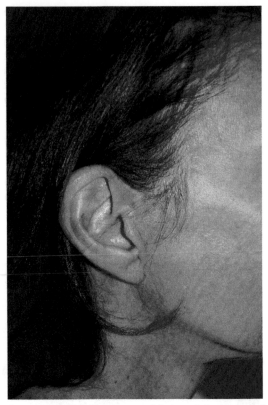

Fig. 16. Well-healed temporal hair tuft incision and post-tragal incisions. This close-up photo shows the patient in **Fig. 15** 12 months postoperatively.

required submental liposuction. The bruising with this technique is usually limited to the skin flap that remains that is posterior to the deep-plane entry point (**Fig. 18**). There were relatively few complications in this series.

- Three patients (1.9%) experienced hematoma: 1 required additional surgical intervention and 2 were managed conservatively with needle aspiration.
- Two patients (1.3%) had temporary nerve paresis (one marginal mandibular and one temporal) that resolved within 6 weeks.
- There were no cases of permanent nerve injury.
- One patient required the removal of one nonabsorbable 3-0 suspension suture because of palpability on the surface. The authors think that this low incidence of suture show is caused by the thickness of the deep-plane facelift flap, but it is acceptable to use Mersilene (Ethicon, Inc, Somerville, NJ) or a Polydiaxonone suture (Ethicon, Inc, Somerville, NJ) as a substitute for the suspension sutures.

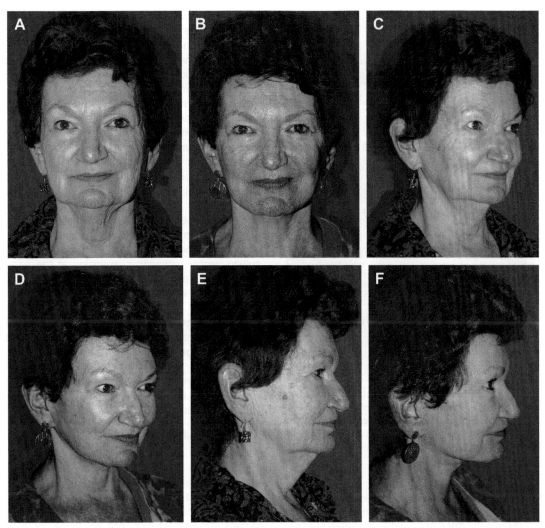

Fig. 17. (*A, C, E*) This 65-year-old woman presented with a turkey gobbler, heavy jowls, and thick platysmal cording and was not a candidate for a MADE short-incision facelift. (*B, D, F*) Eleven months after deep-plane rhytidectomy requiring an extended posterior auricular/occipital hairline incision with midline platysmaplasty. Note the complete correction of the platysmal banding and cervicomental laxity.

Second series of 142 facelift patients Following this initial series, the authors reviewed their experience with the next 142 rhytidectomy patients. Their average age was 57.8 years (range, 36–75 years), and the average length of follow-up was 11.9 months. Of this group, 42 (29%) were not candidates for the MADE technique by preoperative evaluation as described earlier and required a postauricular/occipital hairline incision and a midline platysmaplasty. The authors think that fewer patients were candidates for the MADE technique because they became more stringent with the indications for this technique. Some patients with more significant submental laxity do better with the additional removal of horizontal skin excess and midline platysmal work even when the

preoperative evaluation indicates that they are good candidates. Essentially, the authors became more aware of the limitations of this procedure in older patients with more severe facial ptosis.

- The tuck-up rate for this group of 142 was 3% (4).
- Complication rates in this group included a hematoma rate of 2.0% and 1.4% had temporary nerve paresis (2 marginal mandibular) that resolved within 6 weeks.
- There were no permanent facial nerve injuries in 342 consecutive patients (**Table 1**).

Analysis of vertical vectors in 150 facelift patients The authors also performed a detailed analysis of the vertical vectors applied in the

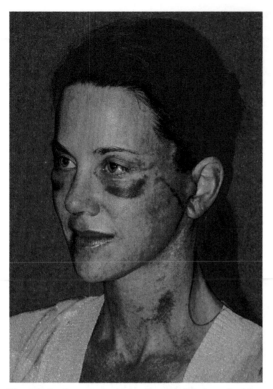

Fig. 18. Patient at 1 week after MADE short-incision facelift. Note limited bruising anterior to the deep-plane entry point because of the fascial deeper plane of dissection. Periorbital bruising is from a simultaneous lower blepharoplasty.

MADE lift procedure in a prospective outcomes study of 150 consecutive facelift patients (300 hemifaces).[24] After complete elevation of the composite skin and SMAS flap, the angle of

maximal rejuvenation was determined for the hemiface. The 3 suspension sutures (3-0 nylon) were placed in the lateral shelf of the deep-plane flap. The flap was rotated from directly horizontal (0°) and moved toward the vertical axis (90°). As the flap was moved, careful attention was given to the submental area, jawline, and midface. The angle that resulted in the greatest reduction of submental laxity and jowling, without flattening the midface (as seen with overly horizontal flap redraping) or creating malar bunching and lateral-facial pleats (as seen with overly vertical flap redraping), was used.

The skin to be excised was measured in situ after the placement of a key tacking suture; all measurements were recorded in millimeters. Standard trigonometry was used to calculate the resulting vector following suspension at the angle of maximal rejuvenation. Skin excision for the cohort overall was 31 mm in the vertical dimension (range, 16–49 mm) and 18 mm in the horizontal direction (range, 9–30 mm). The average angle of maximal rejuvenation was 60° from the horizontal direction (range, 46°–77°).

The angle of maximal rejuvenation was inversely correlated to patient age ($r = -0.3$). The resulting angle was significantly greater for younger patients (aged <50 years, 64°) than for older patients (aged ≥70 years, 54°; $P<.0002$). In the authors' study, 300 hemifaces were lifted. A breakdown of skin excess and angle according to patient age is presented in **Table 2**. Clinical examples are given in **Figs. 19–22**. Calculation of the angles of maximal rejuvenation in each case shows that flap suspension is indeed superoposterior, not posterior, or even posterosuperior. In all hemifaces, regardless of

Table 1 Outcomes and complications for MADE vertical facelift		
Total 323 Patients	**First 181 Facelifts**	**Next 142 Facelifts**
Average age (y)	58	60
Posterior limb incision	15% (28)	29% (42)
Tuck-up rate	3.9% (6)	3.0% (4)
Hematoma	1.9% (3)	2.1% (3)
Temporary facial nerve paresis	1.3% (2)	1.4% (2)
Midline platysmaplasty	12% (20)	13% (21)

Table 2
Vector of facial suspension in MADE vertical facelift by age category

Age Group (y)	Number of Hamifaces	Average Vertical Excess (mm)	Average Horizontal Excess (mm)	Average Angle (degree)
≤49	44	33	16	64
50–59	92	32	17	61
60–69	124	32	19	59
70–79	26	30	20	57
≥80	4	18	14	51
Total	300	31	18	60

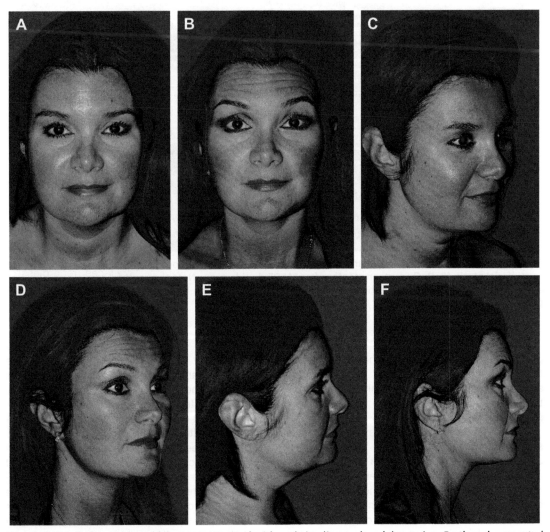

Fig. 19. (A, C, E) This 42-year old woman presented with early jowling and neck loosening. Further, she reported a loss of the heart-shaped contour of her more youthful face. (B, D, F) Thirteen months after MADE rhytidectomy. Note the midface correction, particularly in the oblique view, and the alleviation of all signs of early jowling. The vector of lift for this patient was 74°.

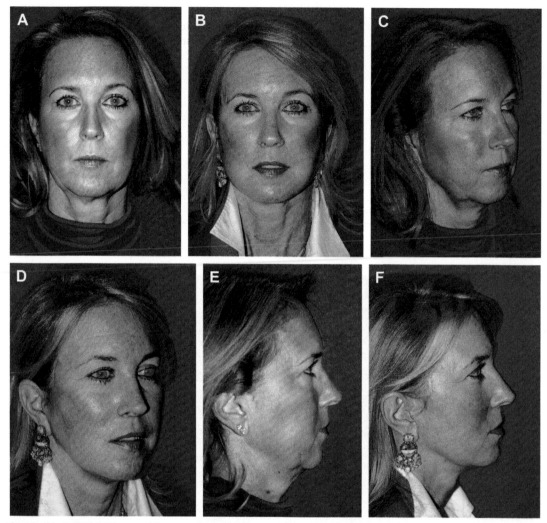

Fig. 20. (*A, C, E*) This 54-year-old woman had significant concerns about her loosening neck and jowls, in addition to midfacial ptosis. (*B, D, F*) Fourteen months after MADE rhytidectomy. Note the youthful cervicomental region and midface volumization with vertical elevation of the deep-plane flap in the cheek. The vector of lift for this patient was 62°.

patient age, this angle was found to be greater than 45° from the horizontal direction. The authors think it is this vertical midface elevation that allows for greater midface rejuvenation in rhytidectomy.

It is worth noting that a previous hemiface study comparing deep-plane and SMAS-lift approaches in the same patient failed to show a significant or identifiable difference in midfacial rejuvenation between sides.[3] The authors think that the lack of midface improvement in this study was not related to the efficacy of a composite/deep-plane technique but rather the angle of the flap resuspension. This study preceded the advent of vertical-vector face lifting, which was

subsequently described and popularized by the MACS lift and derivative operations.[1,20] The release of the midface with a more horizontal vector of tightening (ie, more posterior than superior) does not elevate the midface but simply flattens it, resulting in little midface improvement. When the deep-plane rhytidectomy flap is suspended vertically, the midface is lifted and not flattened.

The authors prefer this approach to midface rejuvenation over fat grafting because it avoids the need of a second procedure during the facelift and also reduces the cost to patients. Further, fat grafting is associated with inconsistent take rates because fat grafts are free nonvascularized grafts.

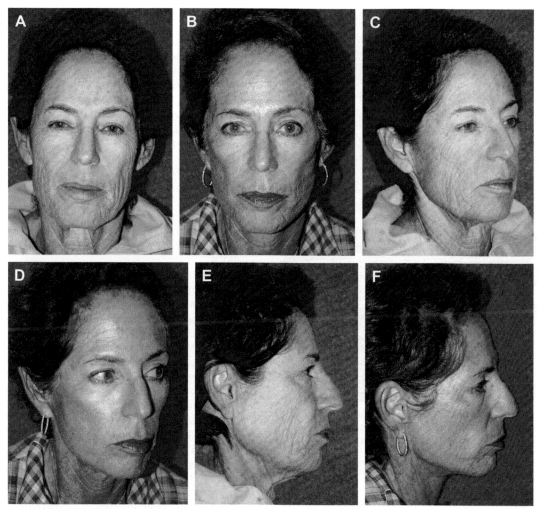

Fig. 21. (*A, C, E*) This 64-year-old woman presented with excessive cervical laxity, jowls, and a devolumized midface. (*B, D, F*) Twenty-nine months after rhytidectomy. Note the complete correction of the platysmal banding and cervicomental laxity. The vector of lift for this patient was 50°.

This inconsistency leads to surgical failures in a high percentage of cases, often requiring multiple sessions of fat transfers with multiple recoveries to patients. The authors have demonstrated a 33% patient dissatisfaction rate with fat grafting caused by graft reabsorption, incomplete graft take, and lack of midface improvement.[25]

CONCLUSIONS ON MADE VERTICAL FACELIFT

The MADE vertical facelift

- Results in a shorter incision
- Addresses the midface, jawline, and neck
- Has a more rapid healing phase
- Has a low rate of complications

- Minimizes the need for ancillary procedures in aging face surgery, including autologous fat transfers for midface rejuvenation and midline platysmal procedures to improve neck results

MADE is the procedure the authors offer for their patients seeking a minimally invasive procedure. The key to the MADE approach's shorter incision (not requiring a posterior auricular/occipital scalp limb) is the vertical vector of the lift. It can be used in most aging-face candidates with mild to moderate rhytidosis facialis, usually in age range of the 40s through the 60s. Poor candidates for this approach include those with more severe facial ptosis and poor anatomy, including retrognathia, low anterior hyoid, and severe platysmal redundancy.

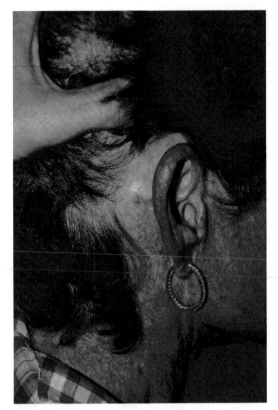

Fig. 22. Note the postauricular incision in the patient in **Fig. 21** is limited to the concha of the ear and does not extend onto the posterior/occipital scalp.

SUPPLEMENTARY DATA

Supplementary data related to this article can be found online at http://dx.doi.org/10.1016/j.fsc.2013.02.002.

REFERENCES

1. Tonnard P, Verpaele A, Monstrey S, et al. Minimal access cranial suspension lift: a modified S-lift. Plast Reconstr Surg 2002;109:2074–86.
2. Chang S, Pusic A, Rohrich RJ. A systematic review of comparison of efficacy and complication rates among face-lift techniques. Plast Reconstr Surg 2011;127(1):423–33.
3. Ivy EJ, Lorenc ZP, Aston SJ. Is there a difference? A prospective study comparing lateral and standard SMAS face lifts with extended SMAS and composite rhytidectomies. Plast Reconstr Surg 1996;98:1135–43 [discussion: 1144–7].
4. Becker FF, Bassichis BA. Deep-plane face-lift vs superficial musculoaponeurotic system plication face-lift: a comparative study. Arch Facial Plast Surg 2004;6:8–13.
5. Prado A, Andrades P, Danilla S, et al. A clinical retrospective study comparing two short-scar face lifts: minimal access cranial suspension versus lateral SMASectomy. Plast Reconstr Surg 2006;117:1413–25 [discussion: 1426–7].
6. Kamer FM, Parkes ML. The two-stage concept of rhytidectomy. Trans Sect Otolaryngol Am Acad Ophthalmol Otolaryngol 1975;80:546–50.
7. Aufrecht HW, Baker TJ. Rhytidectomy: a look back and a look forward. Ann Plast Surg 2005;55:565–70.
8. Tipton JB. Should the subcutaneous tissue be plicated in a face lift? Plast Reconstr Surg 1974;54:1–5.
9. Rees TD, Aston SJ. A clinical evaluation of the results of submusculo-aponeurotic dissection and fixation in face lifts. Plast Reconstr Surg 1977;60:851–9.
10. Hamra ST. The deep-plane rhytidectomy. Plast Reconstr Surg 1990;86:53–61.
11. Kamer FM, Frankel AS. SMAS rhytidectomy versus deep plane rhytidectomy: an objective comparison. Plast Reconstr Surg 1998;102(3):878–81.
12. Sundine MJ, Krestis V, Connel BF. Longevity of SMAS facial rejuvenation and support. Plast Reconstr Surg 2010;126(1):229–37.
13. Jacono AA, Parikh SS. The minimal access deep plane extended vertical facelift. Aesthet Surg J 2011;31:874–90.
14. Brandt MG, Hassa A, Roth K, et al. Biomechanical properties of the facial retaining ligaments. Arch Facial Plast Surg 2012;14(4):289–94.
15. Whetzel TP, Stevenson TR. The contribution of the SMAS to the blood supply in the lateral face lift flap. Plast Reconstr Surg 1997;100(4):1011–8.
16. Meade RA, Teotia SS, Griffeth LK, et al. Facelift and patterns of lymphatic drainage. Aesthet Surg J 2012;32:39.
17. Marchac D, Sandor G. Facelifts and sprayed fibrin glue: an outcome analysis of 200 patients. Br J Plast Surg 1994;47:306.
18. Rees TD, Barone CM, Valauri FA. Hematomas requiring surgical evacuation following facelift surgery. Plast Reconstr Surg 1994;93:1185.
19. Parikh SS, Jacono AA. Deep-plane face-lift as an alternative in the smoking patient. Arch Facial Plast Surg 2011;13(4):283–5.
20. Verpaele A, Tonnard P, Gaia S, et al. The third suture in MACS-lifting: making midface lifting simple and safe. J Plast Reconstr Aesthet Surg 2007;60(12):1287–95.
21. Kamer FM, Markarian A. Deep-plane technique. Arch Facial Plast Surg 2006;8(3):193–4.
22. Matarasso A, Elkwood A, Rankin M, et al. National plastic surgery survey: face lift techniques and

complications. Plast Reconstr Surg 2000;106(5): 1185–95.

23. Jacono AA, Parikh SS, Kennedy WA. Anatomical comparison of platysmal tightening using superficial musculoaponeurotic system placation vs deep-plane rhytidectomy techniques. Arch Facial Plast Surg 2011;13(6):395–7.

24. Jacono AA, Ransom ER. Patient-specific rhytidec-tomy: finding the angle for maximal rejuvenation. Aesthet Surg J 2012;32(7):804–13.

25. Jacono AA, Ransom E. Anatomic predictors of unsatisfactory outcomes in surgical rejuvenation of the midface. JAMA Facial Plast Surg 2013; 24:1–9.

Endoscopic Brow Lifts
Have They Replaced Coronal Lifts?

Hedyeh Javidnia, MD*, Jonathan Sykes, MD

KEYWORDS

- Brow lift • Periorbital rejuvenation • Endoscopic • Minimally invasive • Brow ptosis • Coronal lift
- Pretrichial lift

KEY POINTS

- The advantages and disadvantages of endoscopic versus traditional brow-lifting techniques have not been proved using rigorous scientific studies.
- We have found that endoscopic brow lifting alone or combined with a trichophytic skin resection can be used to achieve excellent brow and periorbital rejuvenation in most patients with minimal complication and excellent longevity.
- Complication rates, outcomes, and longevity of these procedures using different approaches remain to be studied.

RESULTS, OUTCOMES, AND COMPLICATIONS OF THE CORONAL AND PRETRICHIAL APPROACH VERSUS THE ENDOSCOPIC APPROACH

To know and appreciate the advantages and disadvantages of the endoscopic versus coronal or pretrichial techniques would require a prospective, randomized controlled trial to directly compare the sequelae of each type of surgery. Lacking this, Graham and colleagues[1] systematically reviewed the literature published over the last 20 years, since the original description of endoscopic brow lifting. Their search for studies containing original content and no fewer than 20 patients produced 15 articles, which were all retrospective case series. Although these studies show comparable rates of complications and outcomes between the traditional open approaches and the endoscopic approach, a closer study of each article and its methods of determining surgical outcomes and complication rates becomes a convoluted process. The problem in attempting comparisons between the outcomes is that each study used different criteria and outcome measures. These different outcomes measures preclude any type of specific comparison.

The flaw in comparisons made between these studies is highlighted in reported rates of complications such as dysesthesia. Knowledge of the anatomic basis of surgical dissection in a coronal or pretrichial brow lift would mandate higher dysesthesia rates than the endoscopic dissection, but a comparison of studies published to date shows higher dysesthesia rates with the endoscopic approach. One possibility for this is reporting bias. It may be that dysesthesia after a coronal brow lift is often expected and, as such, not reported as a complication in studies involving a coronal approach.

What can be concluded from large series such as that published by Cilento and Johnson[2] is that, when performed carefully by experienced surgeons, each technique can have few

Disclosures: Neither author has any financial or other disclosures with regard to this document.
Division of Facial Plastic and Reconstructive Surgery, Department of Otolaryngology, UC Davis, 2521 Stockton Boulevard, Suite 6203, Sacramento, CA 95817, USA
* Corresponding author.
E-mail address: hedyeh2@yahoo.com

complications and high patient satisfaction rates. In a recently published series, the endoscopic brow-lift approach has been used in patients with male pattern baldness.[3] In another study endoscopic surgery using a small trichophytic incision to lower the hairline was also used in patients with a high hairline.[4] Although endoscopic brow lifting has traditionally not been used for patients with male pattern baldness or high hairlines, these studies show that, with appropriate patient selection, surgical execution, and surgeon's comfort and experience, endoscopic techniques can be used for a variety of nontraditional indications.

Proponents of nonendoscopic (coronal or pretrichial) brow lifts maintain that these are the gold standard procedures for brow lifting. However, there have been no good prospective studies with long-term follow-up including accepted measurement criteria or reporting of complication rates to support this assertion. The question remains, are coronal, subgaleal approaches more efficacious? Do they have better longevity? Or is it just that these are older techniques and surgeons have classically been more comfortable with performing them? These assertions require specific assessment with long-term follow-up studies. Another commonly cited benefit of the open techniques is that they are more efficacious for treatment of forehead rhytids. Forehead rhytids can be treated by myomectomy with endoscopic or open techniques, depending on the needs of each individual patient. At first, all brow-lifting techniques can improve the appearance of forehead rhytids because of the postoperative swelling that accompanies these procedures for months following surgery. Long-term decrease in forehead rhytids is achieved by cutting of the responsible muscles, which can be done with endoscopic or open techniques depending on the needs of each individual patient.

TREATMENT GOALS OF BROW LIFT

The appearance of the eyelid and periorbital region is among the most important aesthetic unit of the face. This region projects a person's mood and is the most frequently watched area by the casual observer. The shape and position of the eyebrows contribute greatly to the overall appearance of the upper one-third of the face. An aesthetic, youthful appearance of the orbit and eyelids requires a well-supported and positioned brow. Ptosis of the eyebrows and peribrow soft tissues is often a part of the normal aging process. The eyebrows may descend below the level of the supraorbital rims, affecting the function and appearance of the upper eyelids (**Fig. 1**).

The goal of the brow-lift procedure is to restore a youthful position to the brow and to improve the aesthetics and function of the upper face and eyelids. When brow ptosis exists and is not surgically corrected, upper blepharoplasty alone can exacerbate brow ptosis and impart a tired or sad appearance to the eyes.[5]

DECISION ALGORITHM FOR DETERMINING INVASIVE VERSUS LESS INVASIVE SURGERY
Patient Selection and Preoperative Planning

Ideal brow position
Ideal brow position varies between gender and race. In men, the brow is generally heavier and thicker, with little arc present, and often lies at or below the level of the superior orbital rim. The female brow is more refined with a club shape medially and tapering laterally. Although ideal brow positions and shapes are often discussed in articles/texts, no ideal eyebrow position or shape exists. The position of the brow is related to the relative contraction of the elevators (frontalis muscle) versus the relative tone of the depressors

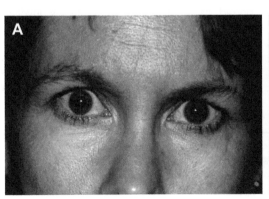
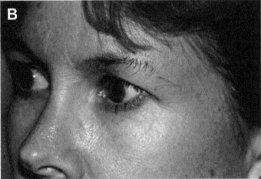

Fig. 1. (*A*) Close-up anteroposterior and (*B*) oblique views of a 40-year-old patient with ptosis of the eyebrows and peribrow soft tissues.

(orbicularis oris, procerus, and corrugator muscles). The ideal female brow should lie just above the superior orbital rim (**Fig. 2**).[6] The medial border of the brow lies on a vertical line drawn up from the alar-facial crease. The lateral end of the brow lies on a line drawn from the alar-facial crease tangent to the lateral canthus. The medial and lateral ends of the brow are on the same horizontal plane. The highest arch of the brow in women is ideally at the lateral limbus or just lateral to it.

The medial and lateral brow should be evaluated separately with regard to their position. The lateral brow often warrants more vigorous elevation, whereas the medial brow is best approached conservatively and should not be overly elevated. We prefer a more conservative medial release to avoid overly elevated medial brows with a postoperative surprised appearance. Our decision algorithm for surgical planning takes into consideration the patients' forehead height and hairline, as well as depth of forehead rhytids and general condition of the patient (**Fig. 3**).

Patient presentation

Many patients present with asymmetry in their brow shape and position. It is the surgeon's

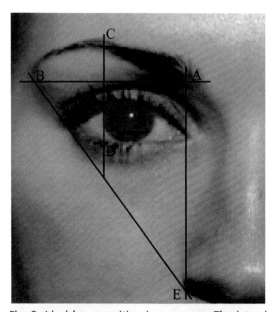

Fig. 2. Ideal brow position in a woman. The lateral brow lies at or above the medial brow (AB). The medial brow begins along a vertical line drawn from the nasal ala (AE). The brow peaks at the lateral limbus of the iris (CD). The lateral brow extends to a line drawn through the lateral canthus to the ala (BE). (*From* Hetzler L, Sykes JM. The brow and forehead in periocular rejuvenation. Facial Plast Surg Clin North Am 2010;18(3):375–84; with permission.)

responsibility to point out these asymmetries and the important effect of brow position on the upper eyelid. It is also important to recognize and communicate why correcting excess eyelid skin and fat herniation fails in improving the appearance of the eyes and upper face if a ptotic brow is not addressed.

Patients with upper eyelid ptosis may often compensate by tonic contraction of the frontalis muscle, which can result in horizontal forehead rhytids. Therefore, it is important for the patient to be in complete repose during preoperative evaluation. To achieve full repose, we ask patients to close their eyes, focus on relaxing the forehead, and gently open their eyes. McKinney and colleagues[7] described certain quantitative measurements to aid in selection of the appropriate lifting technique. They used measurements in a vertical plane from midpupil to the top of the eyebrow and up to the hairline to indicate which procedures and approaches should be used for brow lifting.

Preoperative brow and periocular evaluation can be done effectively by focusing on specific anatomic landmarks. These landmarks include the evaluation of the eyelid including ptosis and levator function, evaluation of the forehead, and overall patient health including overall fitness for cosmetic surgery as previously described.[8]

Eyelid ptosis

If a patient has underlying eyelid ptosis on 1 or both sides, which is best determined by assessing the marginal reflex distance (MRD).[5] MRD-1 is the noted distance between pupillary light reflex and the margin of the upper lid; a distance of 4 to 4.5 mm is normal. The upper lid should lie just below the superior limbus by approximately 1 to 1.5 mm. The MRD-2 is the distance, measured again in primary gaze, between the pupillary light reflex and lower lid margin; a distance of greater than 5 mm is adequate.

Levator function

Levator function must also be measured and recorded when evaluating the periorbital region. This evaluation is performed by holding the brow in position (nullifying the effect of the frontalis muscle) and requesting the patient to first look down and then up. The difference between the position of the eyelid margin looking downward and then upward is the levator function. If a measurement of less than 4 mm is found between maximum down gaze and maximum up gaze, the levator function is deemed as poor; a movement of 5 to 7 mm is fair, 8 to 15 mm is good, and more than 15 mm is excellent or normal.

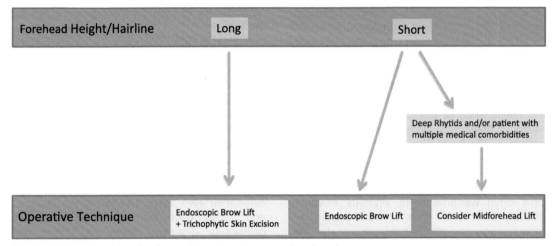

Fig. 3. Decision algorithm for determining invasive versus less invasive surgery.

Upper lid

Upper lid evaluation is to be performed in conjunction with brow evaluation. Analysis of the upper eyelid should include assessment of skin, fat, the height of the supratarsal crease, and aperture opening. If upper blepharoplasty is to be performed simultaneously with brow lifting, it is important to maintain sufficient skin after completion of the procedures to avoid postoperative lagophthalmos. Dermatochalasia is the general term used for the presence of excessive skin and its laxity associated with aging as well as fat herniation. Blepharochalasis is a rare occurrence of unknown cause that occurs typically in women and is manifest by edema, causing decreased elasticity and notable atrophic changes.

Forehead length/hairline position

The forehead may mandate the appropriate brow procedure. Deep forehead rhytids with a high hairline make midforehead lift a reasonable approach.

Patient health

The patient's health may also play a role in preoperative decisions. Unhealthy patients who are not suited for longer surgeries or general anesthesia may preclude more extensive procedures and elect a direct brow approach. In addition, patient psychology and candidacy for aesthetic surgery must be considered.[9]

Preparation for Brow-lift Surgery

Before brow-lift surgery, the use of botulinum toxin helps to eliminate the function of brow depressors, including the corrugator, procerus, and orbicularis oculi muscles (**Fig. 4**). Botulinum toxin use in the forehead elevators (frontalis muscle) is usually not performed perioperatively. The absence of

persistent depressor function promotes longevity of the brow lift and allows readherence of the forehead flap to the underlying cranium. This readherence has been shown to occur within 1 week after surgery.[9] Botulinum toxin injection is performed at least 10 days preoperatively to allow adequate neurotoxin effect. We like to use 16 to 25 units of Botox in the procerus/corrugator complex and 18 to 25 units of Botox in the region of crow's feet/lateral orbicularis oculi.

Patient Positioning

The patient is placed in the supine position with the surgeon at the head of the bed. The monitor for the endoscope should be placed in clear direct view of the surgeon (**Fig. 5**).

Potential Complications and Their Management

Complications of brow-lift procedures vary with the approach and incision used. Possible

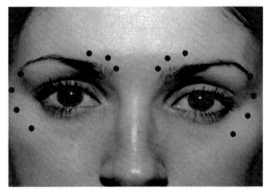

Fig. 4. Sites for preoperative botulinum toxin injection.

Surgeon and Assistant

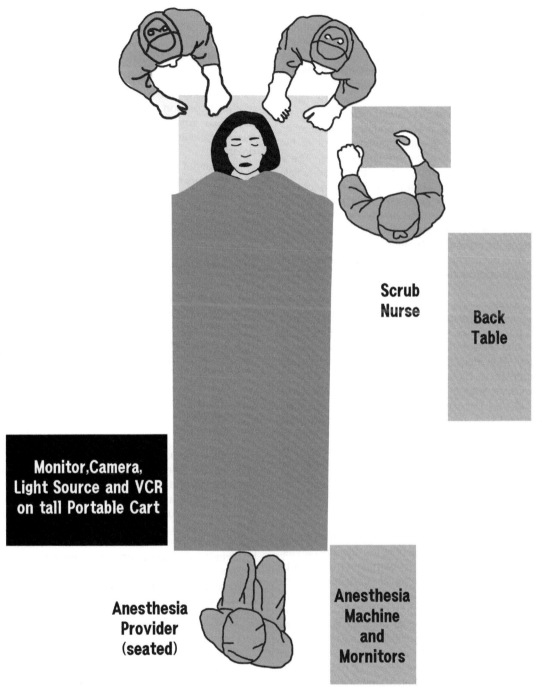

Scrub Nurse

Back Table

Monitor,Camera, Light Source and VCR on tall Portable Cart

Anesthesia Provider (seated)

Anesthesia Machine and Mornitors

Fig. 5. Patient and equipment positioning in the operating room. Papel ID. Facial Plastic and Reconstructive Surgery (3rd Edition). New York (NY):Thieme Medical Publishers, Inc; 2008. p. 233.

complications of brow-lift techniques may include the following:

- Visible scars
- Hematoma/seroma
- Infection/abscess
- Loss of sensation/dysesthesia
- Alopecia
- Nerve damage
- Ocular irritation
- Brow asymmetry

Specific complications of brow-lift procedures often depend on the surgical approach used.

Scars

Scarring is always a concern with brow-lift procedures, and visible scars are produced with the direct and midforehead lift techniques. The scar of the midforehead brow lift is generally hidden in a transverse forehead crease. Unacceptable scars can be improved with dermabrasion or fillers. However, the direct brow-lift scar cannot be camouflaged in a crease and can produce an unnatural change in the superior aspect of the eyebrow giving it a cut-off appearance. These scars could be improved with single-follicle eyebrow hair transplants but, because of the unsatisfactory scar produced, this technique is not often performed. The pretrichial approach to the brow also produces a scar that can be camouflaged by hairstyle. Camouflage of the brow-lift scar is best achieved by the trichophytic or endoscopic approaches.

Alopecia

Alopecia can also occur from either poorly created or poorly closed incisions, including inappropriate wound tension and excessive use of electrocautery. Peri-incisional alopecia can lead to what appears to be a widened scar. In the case of a visible scar by the endoscopic approach, the scar can be excised at a later date. Hair loss around endoscopic scars can make them more obvious and scar revision can be performed to improve the scars by excision the widened scars and reapproximating the hair-bearing scalp. As an alternative, follicular unit hair transplants can be placed in the scar.

Nerve damage

Nerve damage can occur either to the frontal branch of the facial nerve or to the sensory nerves. However, only rarely does permanent damage to the frontal branch of the facial nerve occur. Traction injury to the frontal branch is also uncommon, but, when it occurs, it can last several months. The pretrichial and the coronal surgical approaches are associated with significant transient sensory anesthesia of the scalp and forehead. Sensation typically returns over the course of months, with improvements in sensation starting near the brow and extending toward the vertex, typically with full return of sensation by 12 months.

Brow asymmetry

Before surgery, patients often display some degree of brow asymmetry; intraoperative maneuvers are used to restore symmetry. Postoperative brow asymmetry can result from failure to elevate either brow adequately by inadequate release of the orbital rim tissues. Minor asymmetries occasionally can be improved with strategic placement of neurotoxins.

Immediate Postprocedural Care

We routinely place our patients in a standard face-lift dressing for the first 2 postoperative days. The forehead component places pressure on the operative field, whereas the portion going around the head prevents displacement of the forehead dressing.

The patient is instructed to keep the incision sites dry until sutures are removed on postoperative day 7.

Procedural Approach

The endoscopic approach to brow lifting proceeds as follows:

- First, 3 incisions are made: 1 in the midline and 2 bilaterally at the level of the lateral brow in line with the proposed vector of suspension.
- The incisions are made just behind the hairline and are roughly 1 to 1.5 cm long.
- The initial 3 incisions are made through all layers of the scalp.
- The forehead periosteum is elevated from the hairline to approximately 2 cm above the orbital rim.

Surgical note: care must be taken not to damage the periosteum because it may impair visualization and durability of resuspension.

At this point, a 30° endoscope with a protective sheath is introduced near the supraorbital rim for further elevation of the flap.

The supraorbital neurovascular bundle should be directly visualized and preserved with careful dissection.

Surgical note: 10% of the population has the nerve and vessels exiting through a true foramen, rather than a notch.

- At this point, resection or lysis of the corrugator superciliary muscle may be performed. Some surgeons also perform a radial myotomy of the orbicularis oculi muscle deep to the brow.
- Lateral release of the periosteum is performed at the arcus marginalis at the level of the orbital rim (**Fig. 6**).
- The two temporal incisions are made overlying the temporalis muscle. The position of these incisions corresponds with the vector of pull needed for the desired brow position. Beveling of the incision is performed for follicle preservation.

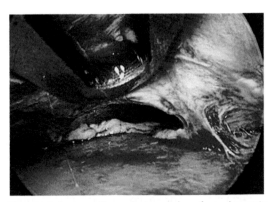

Fig. 6. Intraoperative photograph of endoscopic release of the arcus marginalis.

- The incision is carried down through skin, subcutaneous tissue, and temporoparietal fascia.
- The dissection plane proceeds deep to the temporoparietal fascia, just on top of the superficial layer of deep temporal fascia overlying the temporalis muscle extending down to the level of the lateral canthus.

Surgical note: dissection may be performed under direct visualization. The lateral subgaleal and medial subperiosteal planes of dissection are connected by dividing the conjoint tendon at the superior temporal line. The conjoint tendon connects the superficial and deep layers of temporalis fascia and their medial extension, the pericranium, as well as the junction of the temporoparietal fascia laterally and the galea medially (**Fig. 7**). The sentinel vein may be visualized laterally and is a marker for the frontal branch of the facial nerve. This vein is an extension of the internal maxillary vein and should be preserved.

- Extension of this dissection is performed inferiorly to the orbital rim to ensure full release of the arcus marginalis.
- After complete elevation and release of the brow-forehead complex, suspension is performed bilaterally in the temporal and lateral brow regions.
- The temporal area is first suspended.
- The temporoparietal fascia is suspended to the deep temporal fascia with a 2-0 monofilament absorbable suture.
- Resuspension of the brow and forehead skin is performed next at the incisions made in line with the lateral brow.

Surgical note: the senior author prefers a bone bridge method using a monofilament absorbable suture, such as 2-0 polydioxanone. A bone tunnel may be performed freehand as well as with the Browlift Bone Bridge System (Medtronic Xomed, Jacksonville, FL). Tissue adhesives, the Endotine (Coapt Systems, Palo Alto, CA) device, and microscrews may also be used. Periosteal readherence has been shown to occur within 1 week after brow lift, negating the need for long-term resuspension.[10]

During a brow lift, many have promoted myotomies and myectomies of the corrugator and procerus complex as well as orbicularis and frontalis. This procedure was described in the literature as early as the 1970s.[11] However, the permanent benefit of myotomies has been questioned. The procedure may also have some disadvantages, such as widening of the space between the medial brows and, in the case of a frontal myotomy, depression of the brow.

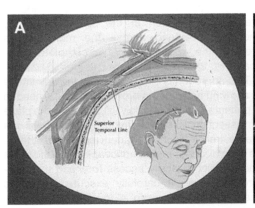

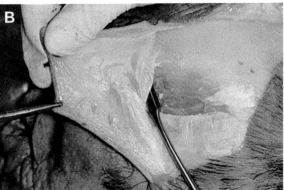

Fig. 7. (A) Release of the conjoint tendon connecting the lateral subgaleal plane and the medial subperiosteal plane at the superior temporal line. (B) Left-sided conjoint tendon at the superior temporal line in a cadaver.

SUMMARY COMPARISON OF TRADITIONAL VERSUS MINIMALLY INVASIVE SURGERY

Nonendoscopic approaches to brow lifting include the coronal, pretrichial, direct, midforehead, and transblepharoplasty approaches. The choice of incision and approach is based on the patient's forehead height and hairline position, the need for myotomy of forehead musculature, and the patient's desired effect and surgeon's comfort and experience with a given procedure.

SELECTION, ADVANTAGES, AND DISADVANTAGES OF EACH APPROACH
Coronal and Pretrichial Approaches

The coronal approach has classically been described as the ideal approach for patients with lower hairlines without significant thinning of vertex hair, whereas the pretrichial approach has been described for those with a high hairline. The coronal approach uses a hidden incision in the frontal scalp approximately 5 to 7 cm behind the hairline, whereas the pretrichial incision is marked 2 mm posterior to the hairline centrally and within the temporal hair laterally. The plane of dissection for both of these incisions is subgaleal, allowing access to the forehead depressor musculature (procerus and corrugator muscles).

It is generally accepted that the more distant the surgical incision is from the brow, the more skin excision is necessary. More skin must be excised for the desired level of brow elevation using a coronal approach compared with the pretrichial incision. In the pretrichial incision, the ratio of the amount of skin incision to the brow lift is 1:5, whereas in the coronal approach it is closer to 2:1.5.

The advantage of the coronal and pretrichial approaches is good access to forehead musculature. In the past, the coronal and pretrichial approaches were preferred because of their time-tested results and surgeons' experience and comfort. The advantage of availability of long-term results and increased surgeon experience no longer applies to the coronal and pretrichial approach because endoscopic brow lifts have now been preformed for more than 20 years and most surgeons are adept at performing them.

Because of their subgaleal plane of dissection, both approaches have the disadvantages of permanent scalp anesthesia, significant postoperative scalp and forehead edema, and ecchymosis. A further disadvantage of the coronal approach is that the frontal hairline becomes elevated by approximately 1 to 1.5 cm. However, this may be desired in a patient with low hairline and short forehead. The disadvantage of a pretrichial approach is a possibly noticeable scar. Beveling of the incision in a posterior to anterior orientation allows hair follicles to grow on the anterior (forehead) segment if the hair follicles are not damaged during the incision, and this can serve to camouflage the eventual scar.

Direct Brow-lift Approach

This simple approach uses 2 incisions at the superior aspect of the eyebrows followed by a subcutaneous dissection plane. It requires minimal undermining and dissection and as such is a useful approach in patients unfit for a more extensive surgery. The advantages of this approach are that it is easily performed under local anesthesia, with or without sedation. Furthermore, the direct approach usually results in minimal edema and ecchymosis. Its disadvantages are that, although minimal dissection is required, there is an increased risk of brow hair loss caused by transection of hair follicles leading to an unnatural, blunted appearance of the brow. It also allows difficult access to forehead musculature. This approach is generally used for elderly patients with multiple medical problems who desire functional improvement without aesthetic concerns.

Midforehead Approach

The midforehead approach may be performed under general anesthesia or monitored intravenous sedation. It is an excellent approach for achieving a precise brow lift with minimal dissection. This approach is particularly beneficial in patients with obvious forehead rhytids and high hairlines and also in those with asymmetric eyebrows, as in cases of unilateral facial nerve paralysis. Incisions for the midforehead lift can be placed in horizontal forehead creases, preferably not at the same level on each side. If creases are chosen at the same level, they should not extend across the midline, thus creating the appearance of a complete linear scar (**Fig. 8**).

This approach is simple and has the advantage of allowing asymmetric brow elevation (as needed in patients with facial paralysis). Because the plane of dissection is subcutaneous, it also does not create transient or permanent scalp anesthesia. Its main disadvantage is noticeable forehead scars and inability to easily access forehead musculature. However, if carefully executed, forehead scars often fade within 4 to 8 weeks. Careful patient selection in terms of possibility of poor scarring (keloid/hypertrophic) and dark-skinned patients is important when choosing this

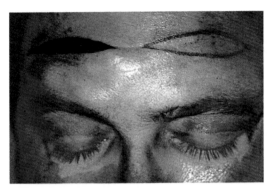

Fig. 8. Placement of midforehead brow-lift incision.

SUMMARY ON BROW-LIFTING TECHNIQUES

In the absence of high-level studies to assess and compare the efficacy of each brow-lifting technique and enable direct comparison between them, all techniques remain relevant in aesthetic improvement of the upper face. Surgical techniques must be tailored to the aesthetic needs and desires of each patient whether they have a high forehead, an abundance of forehead rhytids, or the desire to avoid a large forehead or scalp scar. Furthermore, surgeons must have sufficient experience in, and be comfortable with, their ability to perform the chosen technique with minimal complication rates.

approach. The scar of a midforehead lift is more visible in a young patient, as is the scar of a direct brow lift, making these approaches preferable for rehabilitative rather than cosmetic uses.

Transblepharoplasty Approach

The transblepharoplasty approach provides the benefit of a hidden incision within a natural skin crease. It also involves less dissection, causing less bruising and postoperative discomfort than other methods of addressing brow ptosis. The disadvantages of this approach are that the amount of brow elevation that can be achieved is limited and there may be an increased risk of supraorbital nerve injury and associated numbness. Furthermore, inadvertent stretching of the incision with dissection and fixation may damage the skin at the incision site, leading to poor scarring.

Endoscopic Approach

The endoscopic approach to brow lifting allows minimal, well-concealed incisions that preserve scalp and forehead sensation. There is minimal blood loss and preservation of a well-vascularized soft tissue flap. This approach allows earlier resolution of soft tissue edema and minimal change in the length of the forehead. Although the endoscopic approach has been criticized for lack of long-term results, no good randomized controlled trials exist that directly compare the longevity of the endoscopic approach with any of the traditional open approaches.

REFERENCES

1. Graham DW, Heller J, Kurkjian TJ, et al. Brow lift in facial rejuvenation: a systematic literature review of open versus endoscopic techniques. Plast Reconstr Surg 2011;128(4):335e–41e.
2. Cilento BW, Johnson CM Jr. The case for open forehead rejuvenation: a review of 1004 procedures. Arch Facial Plast Surg 2009;11:13–7.
3. Schipchandler TZ, Sultan B, Byrne PJ. Endoscopic forehead lift in patients with male pattern baldness. Am J Otolaryngol 2012;33(5):519–22.
4. Perkins SW, Batniji RK. Trichophytic endoscopic forehead-lifting in high hairline patients. Facial Plast Surg Clin North Am 2006;14(3):185–93.
5. Fowers RS, Caputy GG, Flowers SS, et al. The biomechanics of brow and frontalis function and its effects on blepharoplasty. Clin Plast Surg 1993;20(2):255–68.
6. Gunter JP, Antrobus SD. Aesthetic analysis of the eyebrows. Plast Reconstr Surg 1997;99:1808–16.
7. McKinney P, Mossie RD, Zukowski ML. Criteria for the forehead lift. Aesthetic Plast Surg 1991;15:141.
8. Hetzler L, Sykes JM. The brow and forehead in periocular rejuvenation. Facial Plast Surg Clin North Am 2010;18(3):375–84.
9. Sykes JM. Managing the psychological aspects of plastic surgery patients. Curr Opin Otolaryngol Head Neck Surg 2009;17(4):321–5.
10. Brodner DC, Downs JC, Graham HD. Periosteal re-adherence after browlift in the New Zealand white rabbit. Arch Facial Plast Surg 2002;4:247–51.
11. Pitanguy I. Section of the frontalis-procerus-corrugator aponeurosis in the correction of frontal and glabellar wrinkles. Ann Plast Surg 1979;2(5):422–7.

The Role of Fillers in Facial Implant Surgery

William J. Binder, MD[a],*, Karan Dhir, MD[b],
John Joseph, MD[a,c]

KEYWORDS

- Facial implant surgery • Cheek augmentation • Malar augmentation • Facial alloplastic implants
- Chin implant • Chin augmentation • Facial fillers • Facial rejuvenation • Facial augmentation

KEY POINTS

- Achieving optimal, long-lasting results in facial rejuvenation requires knowledge of how the aging process affects all levels of the face including the skin, soft tissue, and underlying bone structure.
- Facial fillers and alloplastic implants are 2 methods commonly used to achieve the goal of volume enhancement for rejuvenation of the face. It is important to understand the appropriate use of each technique either as a sole modality or in conjunction with each other to attain optimal aesthetic results.
- Although minimally invasive soft-tissue augmentation procedures such as fillers have effectively improved the midface treatment paradigm, chin augmentation with alloplastic implantation remains the mainstay of treatment of microgenia.

 Dr Joseph demonstrates midface facial filling with Sculptra and discusses his preparation of the materials for tear trough and midface injection in a video that accompanies this article.

TREATMENT GOALS USING FILLERS AND IMPLANTS

Augmentation of the midface and chin with alloplastic implants has been performed with increasing frequency during the past 4 decades and offers a long-term solution for augmenting skeletal deficiencies, restoring facial contour irregularities, and rejuvenating the face.[1,2] Specifically, chin augmentation with alloplastic implantation is the fastest growing plastic surgery trend among all major demographics. The media have also well publicized the advantages of this technique, which has been characterized as "chinplasty" in mainstream magazines, further heightening the awareness of both the aesthetic and psychological benefits of treating microgenia.[3]

In contrast, rates of midface alloplastic implant procedures have increased at a measured pace during the past 2 decades because of the introduction of "less-invasive" techniques such as injectable facial fillers and fat transfer.[4,5] Alloplastic implantation of the chin remains the optimal choice for projecting and repositioning the soft tissue envelope, whereas facial fillers have gained popularity in rejuvenating the aging midface.[5] This more recent reliance on less-invasive surgical and nonsurgical rejuvenation procedures has minimized the key role of the skeletal structure component of the aging midface. However, rather than replacing surgical augmentation techniques, fillers can enhance the ability to use midface implants more effectively to achieve long-term rejuvenation.

No financial disclosures.
[a] Department of Head and Neck Surgery, University of California, Los Angeles, 120 South Spalding Drive, Suite 340, Beverly Hills, CA 90212, USA; [b] Department of Head and Neck Surgery, Harbor-University of California, Los Angeles, 120 South Spalding Drive, Suite 340, Beverly Hills, CA 90212, USA; [c] Department of Head and Neck Surgery, University of California-Harbor, Los Angeles, 9400 Brighton Way, Suite 203, Beverly Hills, CA 90210, USA
* Corresponding author.
E-mail address: info@doctorbinder.com

Facial Plast Surg Clin N Am 21 (2013) 201–211
http://dx.doi.org/10.1016/j.fsc.2013.02.001
1064-7406/13/$ – see front matter © 2013 Published by Elsevier Inc.

The Process and Effects of Aging in the Face

Successful rejuvenation of the aging face entails a multidimensional approach to correct the volumetric changes involving the skin, deep soft tissue, and bony skeleton.[6–8]

- Integumentary changes such as epidermal thinning, decrease in collagen, loss of skin elasticity, and deep tissue volume loss represent the hallmarks of soft-tissue changes in the aging face.[6]
- With advancing age, fat in the malar, buccal, temporal, and infraorbital regions atrophies and produces volumetric changes.
- Fat atrophy extends beyond the subcutaneous level and affects the deeper soft tissues along with the fat pad of Bichat. With continued wasting of the fat pads and loss of fascial support, these areas become progressively ptotic due to gravitational effects.
- The malar fat pad, suborbicularis oculi fat, and orbicularis oculi muscle descend inferiorly, exposing the infraorbital rim, and produce an elevation or "mound" lateral to the nasolabial fold and exaggerate its depth.
- The nasolabial and nasojugal folds deepen, leading to cavitary depressions and hollowness in the submalar regions.
- These changes may also flatten the midface and eventually unmask the underlying bony anatomy.

Over time, the progressive cumulative effects of aging transform the once full, angular, youthful face into a predictably rectangular (or pear-shaped) face, which appears longer in configuration, aged, and fatigued.[8]

Most soft-tissue deficiencies in the aging midface are localized within the recess referred to as the "submalar triangle," an inverted triangular area of midfacial depression bordered superiorly by the prominence of the zygoma, medially by the nasolabial fold, and laterally by the body of the masseter muscle. The aging midface exhibits a "double convexity" curvature caused by weakening of the lower eyelid orbital septum and consequent pseudoherniation of the lower orbital fat pads.[2,8,9]

Age-related morphologic skeletal changes, well described by Shaw, must also be considered during the preoperative consultation. Overall, the aging face is characterized by the resorption of bone along the orbit, midface, and mandible, which leads to a reduction in the skeletal framework and laxity of the overlying skin. The net result of these topographic changes can make an otherwise healthy person appear gaunt.[6,7] These changes are further compounded if the patient exhibits deficiencies in skeletal structure such as a negative vector of the infraorbital rim.

Midface Rejuvenation

The specific goals for midface rejuvenation are to[8,9]

1. Add contour to the upper midface or malar area
2. Restore cheekbone fullness and reduce submalar hollows
3. Soften the nasolabial and marionette folds
4. Reduce the vertical descent of the jowl
5. Smooth out facial lines and wrinkles

Initially, facial rejuvenation techniques were tailored to improve skin laxity alone. In the 1980s, Binder first introduced midface alloplastic augmentation as an independent method for volumetric enhancement of the aging face.[2] Augmentation not only enhances the facial skeleton but also achieves a suspensory effect that redistributes the soft tissue in a more favorable position. By restoring lost facial soft tissue volume and increasing the anterior projection of the area, midface augmentation reduces midface laxity, restores facial contour, and decreases the depth of the nasolabial fold. This result can be accomplished with implantation alone and in combination with a rhytidectomy procedure, whereby augmentation can soften the sharp angles and depressions of the aged face, rendering a more natural postoperative result.[8,9] For these patients, augmenting the bony scaffold of the malar or maxillary regions improve the fundamental base for suspending the facial tissues. This emphasis on volume restoration continues to represent a key contribution to facial rejuvenation.

Later, less-invasive soft-tissue volume restoration techniques such as fat transfer and injectable facial fillers were developed to restore soft-tissue volume loss in the midface.[10–12] Facial fillers are safe and effective; require a short learning curve; and over the more immediate term, are cost-effective for treating mild to moderate soft-tissue volume loss. Numerous specialties have adopted their use in the office setting, and often commercially produced fillers do not require a physician for their administration. Fueled by increased public knowledge resulting from direct consumer marketing and advertising, facial fillers have proliferated in both numbers and types during the past few decades. Originally, soft-tissue fillers such as collagen were used to smooth out superficial changes such as epidermal and dermal rhytids. Over the years, diverse types of fillers offering longer duration times and improved standards of safety and immunogenicity have been introduced to restore volume and contour to the aging face. Fillers are now used to treat nasolabial folds, lips, atrophic scars, the glabella, forehead, and Marionette lines. Thicker versions of hyaluronic acid–based fillers, calcium hydroxyapatite (Radiesse), and biostimulating fillers such as poly-L-lactic acid (Sculptra) and polymethylmethacrylate (Artefill) have also been used for enhancing the volume of the midface, mental, and mandibular regions.[12,13] Relying on minimally invasive techniques as a sole procedure, however, may harbor inherent limitations that frequently result in suboptimal short-lived aesthetic effects. Similarly, alloplastic augmentation as a single modality does not address certain specific sites, such as the tear trough, the skeletonized periorbita, and the inferior extension of the submalar hollowing into the lower third of the face. These represent potential areas where fillers can supplement treatment to achieve an improved long-lasting result. Moreover, fillers may be beneficial in overcoming potential challenges in the perceptual ability to correctly size implants and may ensure optimal volume restoration when conservatively choosing a smaller implant. Longevity in patient satisfaction and volume restoration can be enhanced with decreased amounts of filler during the postoperative period to improve site-specific areas. However, the extent and type

of volume loss contributed by both soft-tissue and skeletal changes must be evaluated individually for each patient to maximize the benefit of multiple treatment modalities.

Chin Augmentation

The goal of chin augmentation is to reposition and rotate a rigid soft-tissue envelope to a more projected position along the inferior border of the mandible. The procedure should optimally expand the chin in a three-dimensional plane while preserving the labiomental sulcus and increase the vertical dimension on the frontal view (**Fig. 1**).

Anatomically, the soft-tissue "chin button" is a dense structural entity that has limited mobility or ability to expand because of the following factors:

1. The amount of subcutaneous tissue between the deep dermis and underlying mentalis muscle is minimal.
2. The mentalis muscle is not only attached to the mandible but also intimately intertwined into the soft tissue of the chin.
3. The anterior mental and more lateral mandibulocutaneous ligaments hinder the leverage

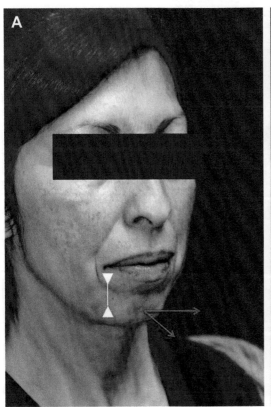 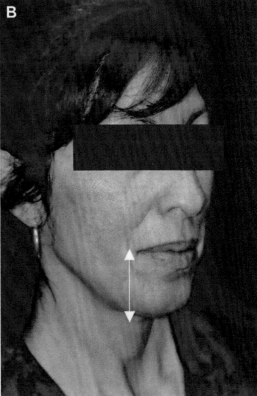

Fig. 1. Chin implant increases vertical dimension by rotation of soft tissue anteriorly (*A*) and inferiorly (*B*).

necessary to expand and dissociate the soft-tissue envelope from underlying bone.

Therefore, treatment with either an alloplastic implant or filler must overcome these factors to improve the aesthetic outcome.[1] Fillers have traditionally been applied to improve a deep labimental sulcus, soften a peau d'orange deformity, and efface the prejowl sulcus.[5] However, all 3 authors agree that because of the aforementioned anatomic inhibitory factors, the projection, rotation, and repositioning necessary for improving the aesthetics of the anterior chin cannot be accomplished with fillers alone.

DECISION ALGORITHM FOR SELECTING SURGICAL VERSUS NONSURGICAL OR LESS-INVASIVE APPROACHES FOR MIDFACE REJUVENATION

A thorough understanding of the aging face and accurate preoperative assessment can guide the surgeon in selecting the optimal treatment and avoiding undesirable aesthetic results. The treatment algorithm depends on each patient's needs, which are dictated by the relative contributions of soft-tissue and skeletal deficiencies.

Filler Alone

In patients with mild to moderate soft-tissue volume loss and minimal midface skeletal volume loss, fillers or fat transfer alone can effectively rejuvenate the face (**Fig. 2**). In addition, fillers can successfully treat site-specific regions involving the tear trough and skeletonized periorbita, as well as mild to moderate inferiorly extended submalar hollowness (**Fig. 3**).

The patients in **Figs. 2** and **3** were treated with poly-L-lactic acid (Sculptra) in multiple soft-tissue planes.

Dilution

The treating author's (J.J.) method includes diluting the product 1 day before injection.

- The dilution solution includes 7 mL of sterile water and 3 mL of 2% plain lidocaine.
- Once the product is diluted, it is warmed to 100°F to deter from the natural tendency of the product to aggregate on the day of injection.

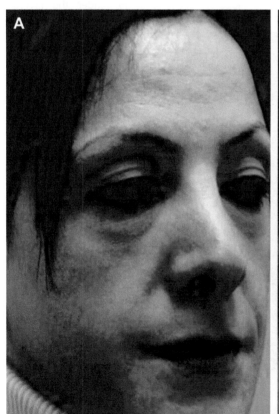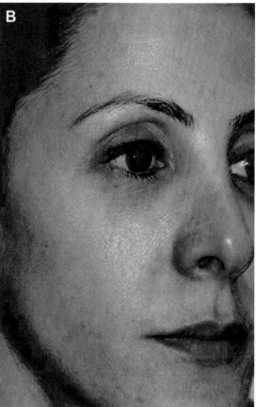

Fig. 2. Before (A) and after (B) correction of moderate loss of soft-tissue volume using poly-L-lactic acid applied to the tear trough, inferior orbital rim, and midface hollow in a case with adequate skeletal structure.

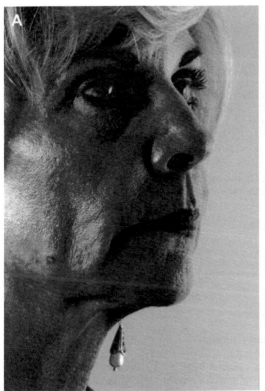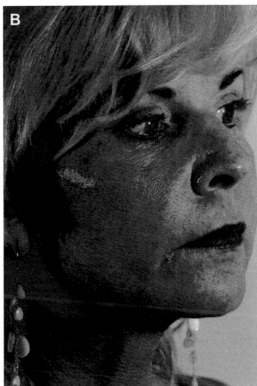

Fig. 3. Patient with adequate skeletal development injected to the tear trough, inferior orbital rim, submalar hollow, and prejowl region before (*A*) and after (*B*) injection with poly-L-lactic acid.

Anesthesia

- Local anesthesia is administered at 2 injection sites: the first injection site is in the plane of the midpupillary line, and the second is slightly lateral to the lateral canthus.

Injection

- The injection sites are approximately at the junction of the thin eyelid skin and thicker midface skin.
- A 3-mL syringe and a 23-gauge (1.5 in) needle is then used for injecting the product beginning at the lateral canthus injection site.
- First, the product is injected in a submuscular/supraperiosteal plane along the inferior orbital rim in retrograde fashion.
- Next, the product is injected superiorly along the lower eyelid in a supramuscular plane to approximately 1 cm from the tarsal plate.
- The product is then massaged superiorly toward the tarsal plate to minimize the needle trauma to this area.
- Next, the needle is placed in the medial injection site and the same injection technique is used to fill the inferior orbital rim, medial lower eyelid.

- A total of 3 mL on each side is injected per session.
- The midface and tear trough region may be treated at the same time by injecting into the dermal-subcutaneous fat junction.

The average patient undergoes 3 sessions during a 4-month period. Patients tolerate the injection procedure with minimal discomfort when injecting in the correct plane.

Treatment of Various Patterns of Midface Deformities with Implants

Recognizing patterns of midface deformity is essential for selecting the optimal implant shape and size to obtain the best overall effects in facial contouring (**Table 1**).

Patients with type I deformities exhibit good midfacial fullness but have insufficient malar skeletal development. In these cases, a malar implant can augment the zygoma and create the appearance of a lateral-projecting cheek bone (**Fig. 4**A). The second deformity (type IIa) is characterized by atrophy of the midface soft tissue and adequate malar development. The submalar depression does not extend inferiorly past the inferior border of the zygoma into the lower third of the face

Table 1
Facial deformity types and recommended treatment approaches

| | Deformity Type | | Augmentation Required | Treatment Protocol |
	Soft Tissue	Skeletal		
—	Mild to moderate loss	Adequate development	Subcutaneous tissue volume in site-specific areas	May use fillers or fat transfer for mild subcutaneous loss, tear trough, skeletonized infraorbital rim/periorbita (thin skin), Marionette lines, and nasolabial folds
Type I	Adequate volume	Malar hypoplasia	Projection over the malar eminence	Conform malar implant: "shell type" extending inferiorly into submalar space for improved contour Minimal amount of fillers or fat may be used adjunctively for asymmetry with sizing, tear trough, skeletonized intraorbital rim (thin skin), and subcutaneous loss
Type II (IIa/IIb)	Submalar volume deficiency (primarily in upper half of submalar triangle)	Adequate development	Requires anterior projection Implant placed over face of maxilla and/or masseter tendon in submalar space Provides midfacial fill	Conform submalar implant Filler or fat for site-specific areas including lower half of submalar triangle if necessary
Type III	Submalar volume deficiency	Malar hypoplasia	Requires anterior and lateral projection; "volume replacing implant" for entire midface restructuring	Combined midface implant (malar-submalar) Fills large midfacial void Fillers alone inadequate to create project necessary and may result in overfilling of product and amorphous facial contour Adjunctive fillers or fat may be used for site-specific areas and sizing issues

(type IIb). The implant must provide a midfacial projection. Type IIa deformities are treated with a conform submalar implant (see **Fig. 4**B). Type IIb is a subtype II deformity involving a subset of submalar depressions that extend into the lower third of the face. This condition is treated either with filler alone or with a submalar implant placed in the submalar deficiency, with filler or fat placed into the submalar extension lateral to the nasolabial and Marionette line. A third variation (type III deformity) arises from combined malar hypoplasia and midfacial soft-tissue volume loss (see **Fig. 4**C). In this deformity, described as the "volume-deficient face," a combined implant (malar-submalar) or the new conform midfacial implant proportionally augments the deficient skeletal structure while filling the void created by midfacial volume loss (**Fig. 5**).

PATIENT SELECTION

The normal aging process commences between the third and fourth decades of life and rapidly accelerates through the fifth and sixth decades. This is consistent with Shaw's finding that statistically significant losses in skeletal volume occurred on average between the ages of 24.7 and 50.2 years.[6] Although prospective candidates

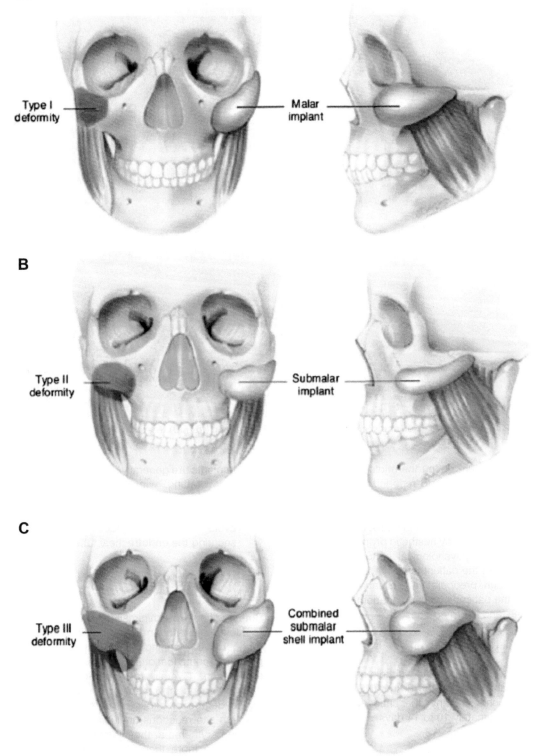

Fig. 4. Implant placement by facial deformity type. (*A*) In type I deformity, malar shell implants rest in a more superior and lateral position over the malar and zygomatic bone. (*B*) Submalar implants for type II deformity are situated over the anterior face of the maxilla. (*C*) For type III, combined malar-submalar implants cover both the malar bony eminence and the submalar triangle. (*From* Binder WJ, Kim BP, Azizzadeh B. Aesthetic midface implants. In: Azizzadeh B, Murphy MR, Johnson CM, editors. Master techniques in facial rejuvenation. Philadelphia: Saunders; 2007. p. 197–215; with permission.)

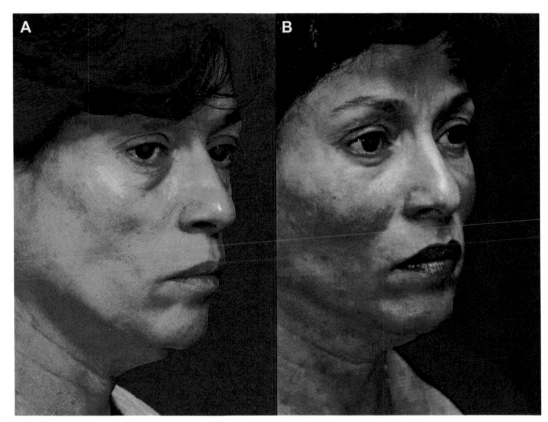

Fig. 5. Patient with soft-tissue and skeletal volume loss before (*A*) and after (*B*) treatment with alloplastic implantation of the midface.

typically present during the midlife or later years, the surgeon's ability to recognize structural and soft-tissue defects and alterations in anatomy plays a critical role in assessing a patient's eligibility for facial rejuvenation procedures. Before proceeding with any aesthetic procedure, assessing both the psychological status and medical condition of the patient is paramount. In addition, a thorough preoperative evaluation should address the patient's goals, management of expectations, and informed consent.

PREOPERATIVE PLANNING

Patients are instructed to withhold aspirin, nonsteroidal antiinflammatory drugs (NSAIDs), herbal supplements, and any other anticoagulant therapy for approximately 10 to 14 days.

PATIENT POSITIONING

- Markings are applied with the patient in the upright position before performing any rejuvenation technique.
- Facial fillers are typically injected in the upright to semirecumbent position.

- Implants are generally placed in an operating room setting, with the patient in a supine position.
- If the patient is intubated, it is important to avoid distorting the facial anatomy when securing the endotracheal tube to the face.

POTENTIAL COMPLICATIONS AND THEIR MANAGEMENT

Both traditional and minimally invasive approaches to facial rejuvenation can benefit from proper preoperative planning to minimize the risk of potential complications and maximize patient satisfaction. Overall, technique-dependent and patient-dependent variables can also contribute to the degree of expected complications. Early injection site reactions, including swelling, bruising, and erythema at the injection site, have been reported in more than 90% of subjects treated with soft-tissue fillers in clinical studies.[14] However, in practice, the extent of superficial trauma depends on the gauge of the needle and viscosity of the filler; more viscous fillers requiring larger needles can lead to greater disruption of the dermal structures, with subsequent capillary leakage, edema, and inflammation.[14] In addition, the location of the injection may determine the extent of local trauma. For example, swelling and bruising can occur more frequently after injections of filler in highly vascular areas, such as the lip or tear trough sulcus. Typically, swelling and bruising after the injection of soft-tissue fillers can persist for 4 to 7 days but may be minimized by advising the patient to avoid aspirin, NSAIDs, and vitamin supplements for 7 to 10 days before the procedure. Hypersensitivity reactions to dermal fillers, particularly those containing bovine collagen, pose a theoretical risk but have been reported in the published literature.[14] In addition to these potential complications, improper technique and/or injection of too little or too much filler can lead to undesirable aesthetic results or lack of longevity (**Fig. 6**). Migration and asymmetric resorption of tissue fillers may also occur (**Fig. 7**).

Catastrophic complications include vessel injury than can result in skin infarction and ultimately skin loss. These complications are minimized when injecting within the correct plane. Injections of poly-L-lactic acid (Sculptra) as described earlier to the periorbital and tear trough region may potentially present with nodule formation, which typically

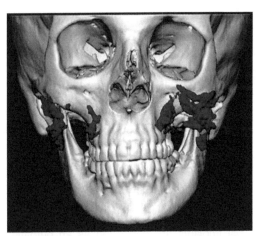

Fig. 7. Coronal computed tomographic image demonstrating calcium hydroxyapatite injected into the midface with migration and asymmetric resorption.

occurs in about 5% to 7% of the treated patients.[9] When visible or palpable to the patient, the nodules may be injected intralesionally with an equal dilution of triamcinolone acetonide (Kenalog), 10 mg/mL, and 5 Fluorouracil. Injections are administered at 30- to 45-day intervals, and most nodules resolve. Surgical removal is not indicated for most cases.

Fat transfer, an acceptable method for remedying medial and central rim skeletonization, can also lead to complications. This approach gained popularity in the late 1990s and was championed by advocates such as Coleman.[10] Long-term follow-up, however, revealed a great deal of variability in the amount of fat that remained viable after harvest and injection, leading to the need for multiple treatments. Moreover, complications such as persistent fat nodules or lumps along the orbital rim occurred postoperatively.[15] Retained fat has also been found to preserve the donor site characteristics, which increases its volume independently and amorphously with substantial weight gain.[16,17]

As with soft-tissue fillers, postoperative edema after implant placement is not uncommon. Approximately 80% to 85% of edema resolves within 3 to 4 weeks.[9] Incorrect placement, insufficient pocket size, or inadequate fixation of the implant can cause malpositioning of the implant; however, the implant should not extrude if proper technique is followed. Other complications include bleeding, hematoma, seroma, fistula, pain, and persistent inflammatory action. Approximately 1% of patients receiving alloplastic silicone implants develop postoperative infections.[16] Infraorbital and facial nerve injury may also occur but is rarely permanent.

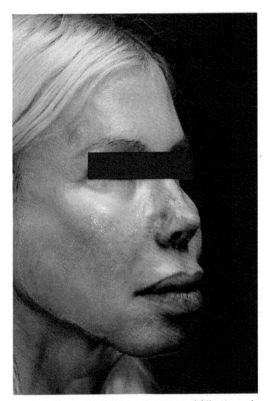

Fig. 6. Injection of excessive volumes of filler into the medial aspect of the midface can result in overfilling of the midface and an amorphous facial contour.

POSTPROCEDURAL CARE AND RECOVERY
Fillers

Typically, no analgesics are prescribed for routine pain management in the postoperative period. The acute edema and erythema may be treated with ice packs for the first 24 hours. Follow-up care is scheduled for 7 days after the procedure. Patients are instructed to contact the treating physician if signs of vascular compromise or impending skin necrosis occur, such as extreme pain, superficial skin changes, fever, or expanding mass.

Implants

Facial implants are performed as an outpatient procedure, and patients usually recover at home. Antibiotics, analgesics, and antiemetics are prescribed, and patients are advised to apply ice packs for 3 to 4 days and to sleep, or rest, with the head elevated. The initial postoperative visit typically occurs on the first or second day and the facial dressings, external sutures, and drains are removed if applicable. Most patients resume routine activity as early as 5 to 7 days postoperatively.

PROCEDURAL APPROACHES
Fillers

The choice of filler used varies depending on the patients' specific needs and goals.

Hyaluronic acids are used for patients who want an immediate but reversible correction with hyaluronidase. Permanent fillers approved by the US Food and Drug Administration, such as polymethylmethacrylate (Artefill), can also be substituted for soft tissue, as well as for skeletal augmentation. However, once injected, it cannot be removed.

One of the authors (J.J.) often injects calcium hydroxyapatite supraperiosteally to augment deficiencies in the skeletal support structure and uses poly-L-lactic acid injected in the dermal-subcutaneous fat junction to replace lost soft tissue in the midface and tear trough. These fillers have biostimulatory properties and confer longer-lasting effects over hyaluronic acid fillers when used for these indications.

Midface Implantation

Surgical insertion of midface implants is a simple, straightforward procedure, which can be performed by an experienced surgeon in less than 30 minutes using intravenous sedation or general anesthesia. The implants are soaked in an antibiotic solution before insertion. During the operation, the surgeon should have access to a variety of implant sizes and shapes and must be prepared to customize the implants if needed.

Chin Augmentation

Chin augmentation using alloplastic implants is a technically simple procedure that releases the anterior mental ligaments and allows for repositioning of the soft-tissue button to a more anterior and projected position. The implant is placed externally through a submental incision or via an intraoral incision along the inferior gingival sulcus. The implant procedure can generally be completed in less than 30 minutes.

The authors typically use the external route via a 1.0- to 1.5-cm submental incision. Technical and aesthetic advantages of the external approach include preservation of the labiomental sulcus by avoiding disruption of the mentalis muscle attachment to the mandible, avoidance of intraoral bacterial contamination, direct access to the mandibular border where the cortical bone is present, limited retraction of the mental nerve, the ability to easily detach the anterior ligamentous attachments near the submental incision site, and the ability to fixate the implant along the inferior mandibular border. Using either approach, however, the surgeon must maintain dissection directly on bone in a subperiosteal plane to create a firm, secure attachment of the implant to the bony skeleton. One may find a condensation of fibrous attachments just lateral to the midline of the mentum. It is often necessary to incise and detach these tendinous attachments to allow dissection to continue along the inferior segment of the mandible. Failure to recognize these attachments may direct the lateral plane of dissection superiorly, placing the mental nerve at risk. Continued dissection laterally also provides an exponential benefit by elevating the deep periosteal attachments of the mandibulocutaneous ligament.

COMPARISON OF TRADITIONAL VERSUS MINIMALLY INVASIVE SURGICAL APPROACHES

Published studies indicate that malar augmentation with fillers can also enhance the upper cheek by secondarily lifting and elevating parts of the lower face. Theoretically, the volume of filler placed into the midface augments and elevates the soft tissue in an anterior-posterior plane. One study of midface hyaluronic acid augmentation used an average volume of 3.9 mL in 72 patients (mean age, 43.6 years) and demonstrated satisfactory results lasting from 4 to 64 weeks (approximately 1–16 months). Midface volume enhancement in cases with ample skeletal structure may in fact elevate the lower third of the face; however, as facial skeletal volume decreases during midlife, augmentation of the soft-tissue plane without skeletal foundation does not allow for adequate suspension of the face and, thus, is more susceptible to gravitational forces. This change produces a deeper nasolabial fold and jowl, as well as aggregation of fillers in dependent areas, and can produce an amorphous facial contour (see **Fig. 6**).

On the other hand, implantation can offer a permanent, more durable option that is completely reversible, and the implant can be removed and replaced under local anesthesia with minimal dissection. Collectively, these benefits make midface augmentation with implants an attractive option for enhancing volume over the long term. This technique also requires a substantially less amount of filler for rejuvenating the aging face over a protracted period.

CONCLUSION ON VOLUMIZING THE FACE

Minimally invasive and facial implantation techniques are safe, effective options for volumizing the aging midface and chin. Achieving the optimal aesthetic result requires an understanding of the multidimensional aging process involving the skin, deep soft tissue, and facial skeleton. Fillers have proved to be a noninvasive option for fine rhytids, nasolabial folds, prejowl sulcus, and the labiomental crease. In addition, facial fillers can also be used for facial contouring in patients with minimal facial bone resorption to achieve midface rejuvenation.

However, the role of alloplastic implantation as a sole modality or in conjunction with either other surgical procedures or minimally invasive soft-tissue augmentation techniques must be considered during the preoperative consultation for both midface aesthetic contour enhancement and facial rejuvenation in patients with skeletal volume resorption. Although chin augmentation with alloplastic implants remains the optimal treatment modality available, using alloplastic implants in combination with minimally invasive approaches may allow the surgeon to address multiple anatomic deficiencies and can promote greater customization of facial rejuvenation techniques.

SUPPLEMENTARY DATA

Supplementary data related to this article can be found online at http://dx.doi.org/10.1016/j.fsc.2013.02.001.

REFERENCES

1. Binder WJ, Kamer FM, Parkes ML. Mentoplasty - a clinical analysis of alloplastic implants. Laryngoscope 1981;91(3):383–91.
2. Binder WJ. Submalar augmentation. An alternative to face-lift surgery. Arch Otolaryngol Head Neck Surg 1989;115(7):797–801.
3. American Society of Plastic Surgeons. 2012 Press Release. New ASPS statistics show "chinplants" are fastest growing procedure. Available at: http://www.plasticsurgery.org/News-and-Resources/Press-Release-Archives/2012-Press-Release-Archives/Chin-Surgery-Skyrockets-Among-Women-and-Men.html. Accessed October 1, 2012.
4. Stallworth CL, Wang TD. Fat grafting of the midface. Facial Plast Surg 2010;26(5):369–75.
5. Lowe NJ, Grover R. Injectable hyaluronoic acid implant for malar and mental enhancement. Dermatol Surg 2006;32:881–5.
6. Shaw RB, Katzel EB, Koltz PF, et al. Aging of the facial skeleton: aesthetic implications and rejuvenation strategies. Plast Reconstr Surg 2010;127(1):374–83.
7. Kahn DM, Shaw RB. Overview of current thoughts on facial volume and aging. Facial Plast Surg 2010;26:350–5.
8. Binder WJ. Facial rejuvenation and volumization using implants. Facial Plast Surg 2011;27:86–97.
9. Schierle CF, Casas LA. Nonsurgical rejuvenation of the aging face with injectable poly-L-lactic acid for restoration of soft tissue volume. Aesthet Surg J 2011;31(1):95–109.
10. Hopping SB, Joshi AS, Tanna N, et al. Volumetric facelift: evaluation of rhytidectomy with alloplastic augmentation. Ann Otol Rhinol Laryngol 2010;119(3):174–80.
11. Coleman SR. Long-term survival of fat transplants. Aesthetic Plast Surg 1995;19(5):421–5.
12. Lambros V. Fat contouring in the face and neck. Clin Plast Surg 1992;19:401.
13. Kim JJ, Evans GR. Applications of biomaterials in plastic surgery. Clin Plast Surg 2012;39(4):359–76.
14. Andre P. New trends in face rejuvenation by hyaluronic acid injections. J Cosmet Dermatol 2008;7:251–8.
15. Cox SE, Adigun CG. Complications of injectable fillers and neurotoxins. Dermatol Ther 2011;24:524–36.
16. Kranendock S, Obagi S. Autologous fat transfer for periorbital rejuvenation: indications, technique, and complications. Dermatol Surg 2007;33(5):572–8.
17. Rubin JP, Yaremchuk MJ. Complications and toxicities of implantable biomaterials used in facial reconstructive and aesthetic surgery: a comprehensive review of the literature. Plast Reconstr Surg 1997;100(5):1336–53.

Fractional CO$_2$ Resurfacing
Has It Replaced Ablative Resurfacing Techniques?

Jesse Kevin Duplechain, MD

KEYWORDS

- CO$_2$ laser • Epidermal ablation • Fractional laser resurfacing • Photodamage
- Postoperative wound care • Pulse duration • Skin rejuvenation • Thermal relaxation time

KEY POINTS

- The fully ablative CO$_2$ laser, the gold standard for skin rejuvenation, is a useful adjunct to facelifting and necklifting surgery.
- Customized skin rejuvenation may include fully ablative and fractional CO$_2$ lasers, fat grafting, facelifting, or any combination of these techniques.
- Fractional ablative laser treatment is associated with the same complications previously seen with fully ablative CO$_2$ resurfacing including hypertrophic scarring, acneiform eruptions, herpes simplex outbreak, infections, hyperpigmentation, prolonged erythema, and contact dermatitis. In the author's practice, complication rates associated with fully ablative resurfacing are no different than recently published rates for fractional resurfacing.
- Increasing the pulse duration beyond the thermal relaxation time of skin (0.8 milliseconds) increases collateral thermal damage, which may result in overlap of thermal zones. This prolonged heating of surrounding tissues may result in a "heat sink" effect resulting in prolonged healing and unexpected complications without improving results. In addition, the greater the treatment density, the greater the overlap, resulting in fractional treatment that may become fully ablative.

 Videos are provided of animation of combined deep fractional and superficial ablative treatments; resurfacing of the upper neck; and resurfacing of deep perioral rhytids accompanying this article at http://www.facialplastic.theclinics.com/

INTRODUCTION

The author of this article uses the pulsed ablative CO$_2$ laser regularly for skin rejuvenation, despite the body of literature describing its adverse effects and the growth of less ablative fractional laser procedures. This decision is based on the gold standard status of the CO$_2$ modality and an innovative posttreatment plan shown in the author's practice to minimize postoperative side effects commonly associated with fully ablative laser resurfacing. Depending on the patient and the severity of the skin condition, the author customizes each treatment, which may also include deep fractional and fully ablative CO$_2$ lasers, fat grafting, facelifting, and any combination of these techniques. A summary of the evolution of ablative pulsed CO$_2$ technology is presented to prepare the reader for a detailed description of the author's approach to skin rejuvenation.

Skin resurfacing refers to the removal of the outer layers of photodamaged skin to stimulate re-epithelialization and collagen remodeling.[1] Aesthetic procedures for resurfacing facial skin may

Disclosure: Dr Duplechain is a funded speaker for Lumenis Inc, Santa Clara, CA, USA. Dr Duplechain is the founder and stockholder of Cutagenesis LLC, Lafayette, LA, USA.
The Aesthetic center, 1103 Kaliste Saloom Road, Suite 300, Lafayette, LA 70508, USA
E-mail address: jkdmd@drduplechain.com

Facial Plast Surg Clin N Am 21 (2013) 213–227
http://dx.doi.org/10.1016/j.fsc.2013.02.006
1064-7406/13/$ – see front matter © 2013 Elsevier Inc. All rights reserved.

be surgical or nonsurgical. Rhytidectomy and blepharoplasty are time-honored surgical techniques to eliminate unwanted jowls, facial laxity, and facial puffiness. Nonsurgical modalities include dermabrasion, chemical peeling, and lasers. Dermabrasion and chemical peeling improve scarring and facial rhytids by burning (chemical ablation) or abrading the superficial layers of skin.[2] Results, however, can be unpredictable because it is difficult to control the depth of tissue removal with absolute precision.

ABLATIVE CO$_2$ LASER RESURFACING

Ablative resurfacing with the CO$_2$ laser is considered the gold standard for skin rejuvenation.[3,4] CO$_2$ lasers, continuous wave (CW) or pulsed, emit light at 10,600 nm and target tissue water, which has a high absorption coefficient at this wavelength. Ablation is limited to the upper 20 μm of skin during any single pulse and residual thermal damage (collateral heating) typically occurs at depths of 0.2 to 1 mm.[5,6] CW CO$_2$ lasers use low-power densities (50 W/cm^2) and gated exposures to successfully reduce wrinkles.[7]

The adverse effects of CW CO$_2$ laser irradiation are multifactorial. Commonly reported complications include the following:

- Persistent erythema
- Acneiform eruptions
- Pustules
- Milia
- Hyperpigmentation
- Hypopigmentation
- Overall lack of satisfaction with the procedure

The degree of thermal damage depends on laser wavelength, irradiance, and duration of exposure.[8] Researchers in the 1980s suspected that tissue could be suitably ablated and thermal damage could be reduced by short pulses rather than long-pulsed, CW CO$_2$ radiation. Walsh and colleagues[8] measured the widths of thermally damaged zones in guinea pig skin after irradiation with pulse durations ranging from 2 microseconds to 50 milliseconds. The 50-millisecond pulse durations produced damaged zones 750 μm wide, whereas the short pulse durations resulted in zones of 50 μm in width.

SELECTIVE PHOTOTHERMOLYSIS

The results of Anderson and colleagues[9] were consistent with the concepts of selective photothermolysis and thermal relaxation time (TRT) of target tissues. In selective photothermolysis, the laser energy is confined to the target tissue for a shorter time (because of short pulse duration) than that required for the laser-induced heat to diffuse to surrounding tissue.[10] The TRT is the time required for the highest temperature rise in a heated area of tissue to decrease to 37% of its peak value.[11] If the pulse duration is less than the TRT of the target tissue, thermal damage to the surrounding tissue is minimized and more desirable thermal effects are achieved. By using pulses shorter than the TRT of the vaporized layer (0.8–1 ms, the TRT of skin), thermal damage zones are reduced to 20 to 150 μm in width.[5,12] The TRT of the target tissue may be used to select the appropriate laser pulse duration time.[13]

Pulsed ablative CO$_2$ lasers permit precise control of tissue vaporization; minimal (controlled) thermal damage; dermal collagen contraction; and hemostasis.[1] CO$_2$ energy instantly vaporizes the surface layer of cells, thermally induces coagulation necrosis of cells and denatures proteins in the subjacent residual layer, and damages cells in deeper zones.[10,14] Similar clinical results can be obtained by scanning a tightly focused CW beam of CO$_2$ energy.[5,12] With this modality, a beam scanner moves the laser spot at a speed that covers the treatment site at an exposure (dwell) time commonly reported as 0.8 to 1 milliseconds, resulting in effects similar to those of a pulsed ablative laser.[6]

THE ERBIUM:YAG LASER

Also an ablative laser, the 2940-nm erbium (Er):YAG device was developed to reduce adverse effects associated with CO$_2$ laser treatment. The 2940-nm wavelength is absorbed 16 times more strongly by water than the 10,600-nm energy of the CO$_2$ laser. Because the penetration depth of 2940-nm energy is only 1 μm, thermal damage is reduced, and ablation is more precise compared with the CO$_2$ laser, whose skin penetration is 20 μm.[5] Research has shown, however, that although wounds heal more quickly and ablation is more superficial compared with the CO$_2$ laser, efficacy of Er:YAG treatment is less when the number of passes and fluences per pulse are comparable with those of the CO$_2$ laser.[14] Dermal collagen remodeling is also less with the Er:YAG laser.[15] Because efficacy of the Er:YAG laser increases with the depth ablation and surrounding thermal damage, pulse duration must be increased to reach the appropriate depth for rhytid ablation and provide some degree of thermal injury.[16] When treatment depths of the Er:YAG laser are increased to those of the CO$_2$ laser, healing times are comparable with the CO$_2$ laser.[5]

ADVERSE EFFECTS OF ABLATIVE LASERS

Traditional ablative lasers have high efficacy but an unfavorable adverse effects profile. Adverse effects of ablative CO$_2$ lasers have been described in numerous reports[1,2,7,17–20] and include the following[2,17]:

- Prolonged erythema
- Pruritis
- Hyperpigmentation and hypopigmentation
- Acne flares
- Milia
- Contact dermatitis
- Infections
- Pain during treatment
- Scarring

With fractional and ablative CO$_2$ resurfacing, treatment parameters must by altered because of the variables associated with each anatomic zone. For example, the risk of scarring is greater in the neck, chest, and extremities than in the face because these nonfacial areas have fewer pilosebaceous units than the face.[21] The depth of the epidermis and dermis vary significantly even within specific facial zones and must be considered to minimize the risks previously discussed.

Nonablative lasers were developed to further reduce adverse effects of rejuvenation procedures. Although nonablative laser treatment stimulates collagen remodeling in the dermis and improves clinical manifestations of photodamage, efficacy is unpredictable and usually less than that of ablative lasers.[22,23]

FRACTIONAL PHOTOTHERMOLYSIS

To address the adverse effects of ablative lasers and the limited efficacy of nonablative lasers, the concept of fractional photothermolysis (FP) was developed. With this technology, the laser beam, rather than completely vaporizing a layer of superficial tissue, creates an array of microscopic wounds at specific depths of the skin with controlled collateral damage to the surrounding tissue. The result is microablation, tissue contraction, neocollagenesis, and rapid healing caused by small wounds and the short migration distances for keratinocyte during re-epithelialization.[10,15] The first FP device was the nonablative 1500-nm erbium glass laser.[15] It soon became apparent that patients needed multiple successive treatments at 3- to 4-week intervals to achieve clinical results comparable with those of a single treatment with an ablative laser.[1,21]

With the success of the nonablative fractional laser came the development of an ablative fractional resurfacing CO$_2$ laser whose encouraging histologic and clinical effects have been reported.[24] Reilly and colleagues[25] recently reported upregulation of matrix metalloproteinases after ablative fractional resurfacing CO$_2$ laser, similar to the molecular alterations observed after fully ablative CO$_2$ laser resurfacing.[26] The fractional CO$_2$ laser combines FP with the ablative 10,600-nm wavelength to thermally ablate a fraction of the skin while carefully heating the surrounding tissue, which after treatment "repopulates" the ablated columns of tissue.[4] Hantash and colleagues[24] showed that collagen remodeling occurred for at least 3 months after treatment.[3] These authors and others subsequently demonstrated that the ablative fractional resurfacing CO$_2$ laser device also tightened skin and improved texture more than that observed with the original nonablative FP devices.[3] Histologic evidence showed that wound repair and neocollagenesis also occur.[4,21,27,28]

ADVERSE EFFECTS OF FRACTIONAL LASERS

Compared with traditional ablative resurfacing devices, reepithelialization after Ablative Fractional Treatment is more rapid, infections are less frequent, duration for posttreatment skin care is shorter, fewer acneiform eruptions occur, and the duration of postoperative erythema is shorter.[3] Fractional laser treatments, however, are not without risk. Avram and coworkers[29] observed hypertrophic scarring of the neck in five patients referred to them after fractional laser treatment. These authors speculated that the scarring may have been caused by reduced wound healing capacity (ie, because of fewer pilosebaceous units for reepithelialization and fewer cutaneous vessels) of the neck compared with the face; facelifting and necklifting procedures that may have produced a "subtle fibrosis" that would have adversely affected the cutaneous blood vessels; and plastic surgery that may have placed underprivileged neck skin on facial sites. They suggested that treating physicians closely monitor posttreatment wound care to minimize adverse effects.

In a retrospective study of 374 patients who received a total of 490 treatments with a deep fractional CO$_2$ laser, Shamsaldeen and colleagues[4] reported adverse events in 16.8% of patients and in 13.6% of treatments of the face, neck, chest, arms, abdomen, and back. Adverse events in order of decreasing frequency included the following:

- Acneiform eruptions, 5.3%
- Herpes simplex outbreak, 2.2%
- Bacterial infections, 1.8%

- Yeast infections, 1.2%
- Hyperpigmentation, 1.2%
- Erythema persisting longer than 1 month, 0.85%
- Contact dermatitis, 0.8%

In a similar study with the fractionated CO_2 laser, Campbell and Goldman[21] reviewed records of 287 patients who received 373 treatments. Adverse effects were recorded in 13.9% of patients and 12.6% of treatments. These effects included the following:

- Allergic or contact dermatitis, 4.6%
- Acneiform breakout, 3.5%
- Prolonged erythema, 1.1%
- Herpes simplex virus outbreaks, 1.1%

The risk of adverse events increased when three consecutive treatments were given to multiple body sites.

Adverse effects have also been found with the 1500-nm erbium doped fractional laser.[30] In their review of 961 successive treatments in 422 patients treated on the face, neck, chest, and hands, complications were observed in 7.6% of treatments. Adverse effects included the following:

- Acneiform eruptions, 1.87%
- Herpes simplex virus outbreaks, 1.77%
- Erosions, 1.35%
- Postinflammatory hyperpigmentation, 0.73%
- Prolonged erythema, 0.83%
- Prolonged edema, 0.62%
- Dermatitis, 0.21%
- Impetigo, 0.10%
- Purpura, 0.10%

THE ABLATIVE CO_2 LASER REVISITED

The availability of these different treatment options enables physicians to customize treatment, depending on the severity of photodamage and the downtime the patient can tolerate. With modern lasers treatment parameters can be more easily controlled and tailored to the needs of each patient.

The author prefers to use the ablative pulsed CO_2 laser over other modalities for skin rejuvenation. The scientific evidence is clear that the fully ablative CO_2 laser is the most effective in creating the desired effect in skin rejuvenation for the following reasons: (1) greater long-term wound contraction and fibroplasia per micrometer depth of injury compared with the Er:YAG laser[7]; (2) superior clinical improvement after equivalent-depth dermal wounding with the Er:YAG laser[11];

(3) greater posttreatment neocollagenesis with the pulsed CO_2 laser compared with the Er:YAG or scanned CO_2 modalities[31]; and (4) a study of quantitative molecular changes in dermal remodeling after treatment of photodamaged forearm skin with a pulsed CO_2 laser showed increased production of messenger RNA for type I procollagen, type III procollagen, interleukin-1β, tumor necrosis factor-α, transforming growth factor-β1, and matrix metalloproteinases-1, -3, -9, and -13. Levels of fibrillin and tropelastin were also observed after treatment.[26] These molecular changes during wound healing were reproducible and resulted in changes in dermal structure of the treated areas.

The treatment conditions necessary to optimize clinical benefits and minimize adverse effects with the ablative CO_2 laser can be understood from the following considerations.[6] The energy needed to ablate skin tissue without charring is approximately 2500 J/cm^3. This amount of energy must be delivered to the targeted tissue for duration equal to or less than the TRT of the skin. Delivery of energy must stop "on time" to minimize transfer of heat to the underlying tissue and prevent charring. When prolonged dwell times are used, superheating of adjacent tissues occurs, which may result in prolonged erythema, extended healing times, and dismay by physician and patient.

The equations describing the energy and pulse duration needed to ablate the uppermost layer with minimal injury to underlying tissue are beyond the scope of this article but may be summarized as follows[6]:

- The heat of vaporization for water is 2260 J/g, which is numerically close to the 2500 J/cm^3 to ablate skin tissue without charring.
- For tissue ablation to occur, the applied fluence must be 2500/α, where α = 500/cm, the absorption coefficient of water at 10,600 nm.
- The quotient, 5 J/cm^2, is the pulse fluence to ablate the uppermost layer of tissue.
- To minimize thermal injury to underlying tissue, the 5 J/cm^2 fluence must be delivered in a short pulse.
- The optical penetration depth is limited to 20 μm because much of the incident radiation is absorbed by water.
- The TRT for the CO_2-heated superficial layer under these conditions is calculated to be approximately 0.8 milliseconds.
- To completely ablate the uppermost 20-μm thick layer of tissue with minimal controlled thermal injury to underlying tissue, at least 5 J/cm^2 fluence must be delivered with a pulse duration of 0.8 milliseconds or less.

POSTTREATMENT CARE

The use of ablative laser skin rejuvenation would be more widespread if posttreatment adverse events were reduced. A perfluorocarbon suspension has been shown to improve recovery from second-degree burns and partial-thickness wounds.[32] These authors also demonstrated upregulation of Type I and Type III collagen expression and increased levels of vascular endothelial growth factor, which stimulates angiogenesis.

The authors of the present report conducted a preliminary study to evaluate the potential use of a perfluorodecalin (PFD) emulsion (Cutagenix; Cutagenesis LLC, Lafayette, LA) as an aftercare product. Patients were placed into two groups and both underwent facial CO$_2$ laser resurfacing.

Group A patients underwent fractional ablative resurfacing followed by application of Aquaphor (Beiersrdorf, Inc, Wilton, CT) immediately after treatment and for 24 hours and PFD emulsion for the next 6 days. Patients received prophylactic antiviral therapy and a broad-spectrum antibiotic for 5 days after laser treatment. Group B patients underwent combined deep fractional and fully ablative resurfacing followed by application of PFD emulsion for 7 consecutive days. Patients received prophylactic antiviral therapy (acyclovir, 500 mg) on the day of the procedure and twice daily for the next 5 days. Group B patients received no prophylactic antibiotics.

Group A patients (who used Aquaphor and PFD emulsion) had a 11-fold increase in milia compared with Group B, who used only the PFD emulsion. Neither group experienced infection nor delay in expected healing times of 1 week.

This early trial has led the author to use the PFD emulsion after all laser resurfacing procedures. Current postoperative care includes twice daily showers, application of antibiotic ointment along incision sites, PFD emulsion three times daily over all treated areas, and cool compresses continuously throughout the healing period to help prevent desiccation of the skin after removal of the epidermis. The complete study is the subject of a separate report submitted for publication.

ARE FRACTIONAL ABLATIVE LASERS COMPLETELY SAFE?

Fractionated and fully ablative CO$_2$ resurfacing are safe procedures when careful intraoperative treatment plans are followed and postprocedure adverse events are minimized. Two recent reports[29,33] describing adverse events after ablative fractional resurfacing of the neck and face demonstrate the importance of intraoperative and postprocedure care, even with this modality. Although standardized treatment protocols offer guidelines for ablative fractional resurfacing, adverse events may still occur, even when the procedures are performed by qualified and experienced physicians. The authors of the present report believe that adverse events are probably the aggregate result of a desire to achieve exceptional clinical outcomes through aggressive laser skin resurfacing treatments coupled with the variability and unpredictability of skin recovery and wound healing that occurs in lasered skin.

Adverse effects with fractional CO$_2$ laser devices have been reported[4,21,29] but definitive explanations for why these effects occur are lacking. The author of the present report uses the pulsed fully ablative CO$_2$ laser regularly for skin rejuvenation despite the growth of less ablative fractional laser procedures with side effects and complications comparable with published data for fractional CO$_2$ resurfacing. This section describes in detail the theoretical reasons why fractional ablative devices may not be as safe as commonly thought; the arguments are based on the role of pulse duration and power in determining how the laser beam interacts with skin tissue.

The goal of skin resurfacing is to achieve ablation with controlled and quantifiable thermal damage to the surrounding (nonablated) tissue. Walsh and colleagues[8] showed that in guinea pig skin, pulse duration is a major factor in determining the amount of this collateral thermal damage associated with CO$_2$ laser treatment. **Fig. 1** illustrates the effects of progressively longer pulse durations on the spread of thermal damage during treatment with a fractional CO$_2$ laser. In each illustration the pulse energy is 30 mJ and the spot size is 120 μm. The pulse durations increase from left to right (0.080, 0.300, 0.500, and 1.200 milliseconds). When the pulse duration is 0.080 milliseconds (equal to or less than the TRT of skin), the zone of thermal damage is narrow, resulting in an accurate and predictable density. As the pulse duration increases to 0.300 the thermal damage zone becomes wider. The increases to 500 and 1.200 milliseconds represent low-power lasers (40- and 20-W, respectively) resulting in unexpected increases in thermal zone damage. These increases in the thermal zone create a wound that was thought to be fractional, but actually has become a wound with continuous thermal zones. These continuous thermal zones may be the cause of unexpected and prolonged wound healing and one potential cause of complications, such as scarring. Understanding this key concept of density as it relates to power and pulse width is paramount to ablative resurfacing.

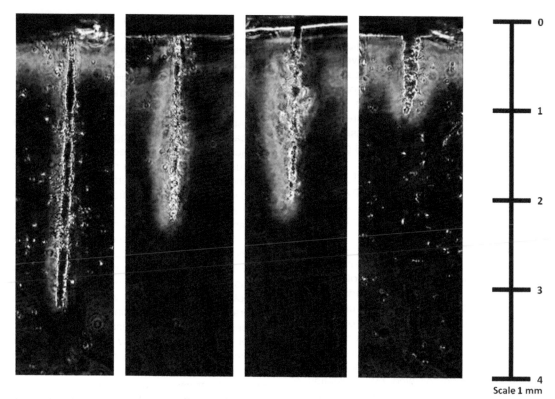

Fig. 1. The effects of progressively longer pulse durations (*left to right*) on the spread of thermal damage during treatment with a fractional CO_2 laser. In each illustration the pulse energy is 30 mJ and the spot size is 120 µm. (*Courtesy of* Lumenis Inc, Santa Clara, CA.)

Fig. 2 shows the wound pattern obtained at varied pulse durations. Each pulse was a 30-mJ pulse, but duration was varied to achieve equivalent energy. As the pulse duration increases, the diameter of ablation and the collateral thermal damage are increased. Although the ablative zones remain fractional, significant overlap of the thermal zone occurs, creating a larger than

Fractional CO_2 Lasers – Pulsed or CW

UltraPulse Wave   SuperPulse Wave   Continuous Wave

Zone of ablation   Char caused by overheating

Narrow zone of thermal damage

Zone of thermal damage

Wide zone of thermal damage

Fig. 2. The wound pattern obtained at varied pulse durations. Each pulse has the same energy, but pulse duration is varied (*left to right*) to achieve the necessary energy. (*Courtesy of* Lumenis Inc, Santa Clara, CA.)

expected wound. The observed increase in thermal and ablative zones with pulse duration is not specific to fractional, but also occurs with ablative resurfacing. One must consider this concept when planning resurfacing because the unexpected increases in ablative and thermal zones that occur as a result of this phenomenon are likely the source of many untoward complications. These considerations offer a plausible explanation of the results shown in **Figs. 3** and **4**. In **Fig. 3**, the patient is shown before and 1 week after treatment with a fully ablative, nonfractional CO$_2$ laser at 100-μm penetration depth. Because the laser is fully ablative, the treatment density is 100%. The same patient is shown in **Fig. 4**, before and 1 week after treatment with a lower-energy fractional laser at 25% density, 450-μm penetration depth. Note also that the spot size was smaller (120 vs 1300 μm) and the pulse duration longer (3 vs 0.25 milliseconds) in the fractionated treatment (see **Fig. 4**) compared with the fully ablative treatment (see **Fig. 3**). In **Fig. 4** the posttreatment skin shows widespread irritation and erythema compared with the occasional irritation and mild erythema in the same patient in **Fig. 3**. This unique comparison of fully ablative and fractional

resurfacing results of the same patient exemplifies the concept of potential delays in wound healing and lack of aesthetic results when certain parameters are exceeded, mainly pulse durations longer than 1 millisecond when ablative thresholds cannot be met. This example shows the low-energy fractional treatment was actually more damaging because the collateral thermal damage zones were greater as a result of pulse durations exceeding the TRT in skin and the resulting overlap of thermal damage zones (**Fig. 5**). This relative "overtreatment" occurred despite the lower energy, smaller spot size, and lower density and of the fractionated laser compared with the fully ablative laser. These effects may explain why patients undergoing fractional laser treatment may experience unexpected complications after treatment.

The foregoing considerations suggest that a better understanding of tissue interaction and the requirements to safely ablate human skin must occur to prevent untoward complications. By applying these concepts to fully ablative and fractional resurfacing, better outcomes for patients may occur. With the dogma that fully ablative CO$_2$ resurfacing provides better wrinkle reduction than

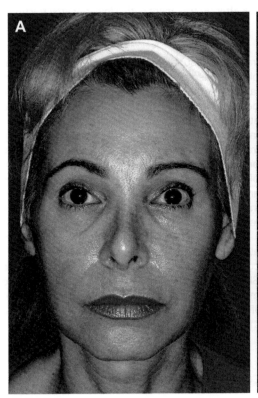 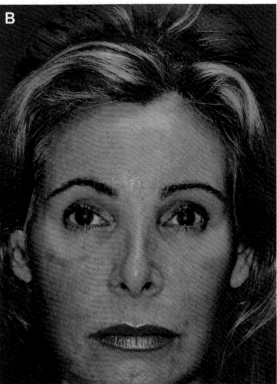

Fig. 3. A 56-year-old woman before (*A*) and 1 week after (*B*) treatment with a fully ablative, nonfractional CO$_2$ laser at 100-μm penetration depth.

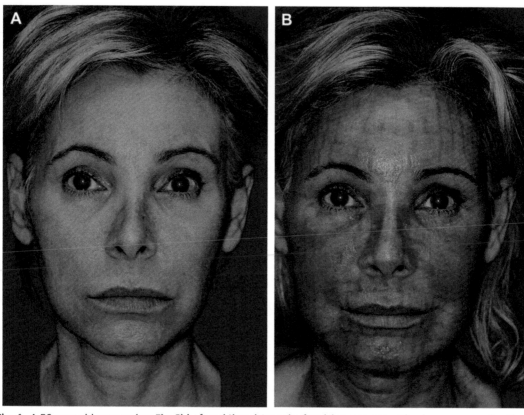

Fig. 4. A 56-year-old woman (see Fig. 3) before (*A*) and 1 week after (*B*) treatment with a lower-energy fractional CO_2 laser at 25% density and 450-µm penetration depth.

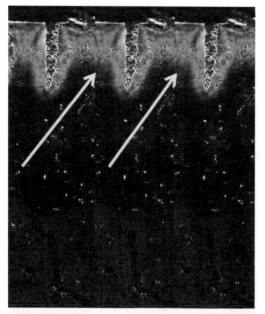

Fig. 5. In each photograph the pulse duration exceeds the thermal relaxation time of the skin, resulting in overlap of thermal damage zones and increased collateral damage to skin. (*Courtesy of* Lumenis Inc, Santa Clara, CA.)

fractional resurfacing, the author has simply applied the discussed concepts to fully ablative resurfacing. By removing the epidermis and part of the dermis with a fully ablative technique, the required structures for reepithelialization remain intact. Certainly, there are cases where both or only deep fractional resurfacing can be used, but care must be taken to minimize overtreatment. Clinical examples are shown in **Figs. 6** and **7**. Video 1 provides animation of combination treatment with deep fractional resurfacing and superficial ablative resurfacing.

The author has taken the foregoing considerations into account in developing treatment protocols for rejuvenating the skin of the face and neck. Skin rejuvenation should be incorporated into most or all of aging face procedures because facelift alone does not address age-related changes to the skin.

FACELIFT SURGERY IN COMBINATION WITH CO_2 LASER RESURFACING

Before 1998, the author performed facelifts using skin flaps and the Superficial Muscular Aponeurotic

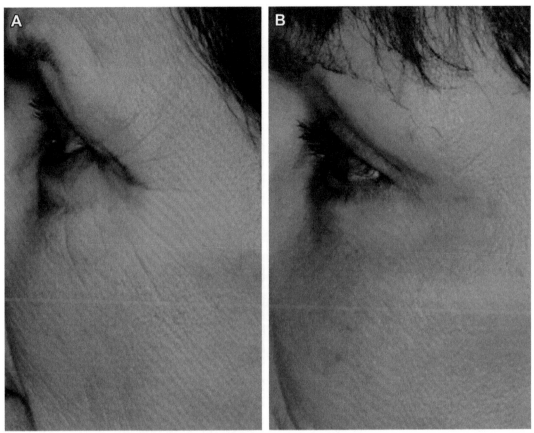

Fig. 6. A 54-year-old woman before (*A*) and 3 months after treatment (*B*) of the eyelids with a fractional CO$_2$ laser.

System (SMAS) imbrication technique. The perioral area was sometimes resurfaced after surgery with lasers or chemical peels, but skin flaps were not resurfaced. Since 1998 the author has performed only deep plane facelifts. For the neck, deep plane surgery has involved wide subcutaneous undermining, whereas for the face, elevation of the subcutaneous layer along with sub-SMAS dissection and elevation are required. Forehead rejuvenation is accomplished by standard subperiosteal endoscopic techniques. Surgery with these planes of dissection raised the possibility that additional benefit could be gained by treatment with a fully ablative CO$_2$ laser, the time-honored gold standard for laser resurfacing. In 2005, the author began to experiment with superficial 1.3-mm spot size fractional CO$_2$ laser resurfacing over skin flaps involving the face and neck (**Fig. 8**). Video 2 shows resurfacing of the upper neck. Because early trial cases provided encouraging results, and without skin loss or scarring, the author elected to proceed with more traditional fully ablative resurfacing. The author has since found that in conjunction with facelifts and necklifts, fully ablative and fractional

CO$_2$ lasers are reliable, results are predictable, and treatment parameters are based on skin depth and tolerance.

The author currently performs CO$_2$ laser resurfacing in all facelift and necklift surgeries. The growing interest in complete facial rejuvenation in which volume is restored, lifting is completed, and skin rejuvenation is achieved has led to a significantly higher level of satisfaction in the author's practice (**Figs. 9** and **10**). Deep plane facelift surgery is followed by fat grafting and CO$_2$ laser resurfacing in all suitable patients. This combination is performed in approximately 95% of the author's facial rejuvenation patients. Post-treatment hypopigmentation, scarring, or loss of skin has not been observed. Physicians should note, however, that fully ablative superficial skin resurfacing is not a replacement for facelift or necklift surgery. Currently, the author does not perform deep fractional resurfacing over undermined neck or facial skin. The depth of superficial resurfacing is defined by the anatomic location within the face or neck and typically involves an ablative effect on approximately two-thirds of the

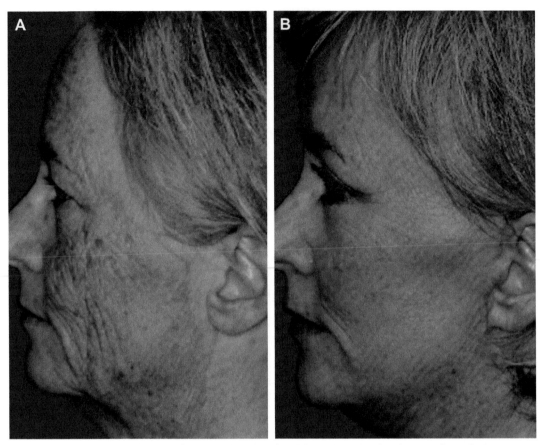

Fig. 7. A 53-year-old woman before (*A*) and 4 months after (*B*) treatment with a fractional CO$_2$ laser.

epidermis and thermal injury effect on the remaining one-third of the epidermis. The overall result is that the entire epidermis experiences a combination effect. The "shrink wrap" effect of

Fig. 8. A 53-year-old woman 3 weeks after necklift surgery. The skin above the top cervical crease was treated with a fully ablative CO$_2$ laser and the skin below the crease was not treated. The treated upper neck skin is much smoother than the untreated skin of the lower neck.

the laser provides additional tightening once the facelift is performed, and helps prevent a stretched or pulled look.

COMBINATION TECHNIQUES
Upper Facial Rejuvenation

For the upper facial rejuvenation my current surgical technique includes endoscopic browlift or lateral browlift with absorbable fixation, and upper lid blepharoplasty with muscle preservation. Lower eyelid blepharoplasty with muscle suspension and canthopexy or lateral retinacular suspension is performed when appropriate. The amount of excess skin is evaluated and the necessary amount of skin is removed. More conservative techniques with a pinch excision are currently used as separate skin and muscle flaps seemed to add an unnecessary risk because lower eyelid epidermal tissue is extremely thin. Lid laxity should be evaluated and canthopexy or canthoplasty should be performed if necessary. Superficial resurfacing is appropriate in lower eyelid surgery, but care must be taken to avoid ectropion.

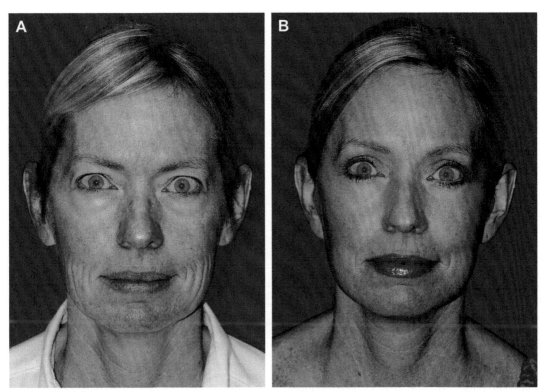

Fig. 9. A front view of a 48-year-old woman before (*A*) and 3 months after (*B*) undergoing deep-plane facelift surgery followed by fat grafting and CO$_2$ laser resurfacing.

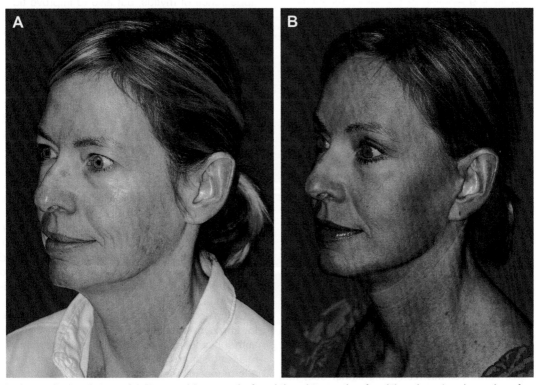

Fig. 10. A diagonal view of a 48-year-old woman before (*A*) and 3 months after (*B*) undergoing deep-plane face-lift surgery followed by fat grafting and CO$_2$ laser resurfacing.

The upper eyelid is treated at 40 μm depth, 80% density, and a 1.3-mm spot size. The lower eyelid is treated at 53 μm, 80% density, and a 1.3-mm spot size. Most of the epidermis is removed and penetration into the reticular dermis and subcutaneous tissue is to be avoided. A clinical example is shown in **Fig. 6**.

Facelift and Necklift

For facelift and necklift surgery, submental platysmaplasty and, when indicated, partial digastric resection or partial submandibular gland resection along with subplatysmal fat resection are performed.

When rejuvenating the neck, physicians should use the laser as an adjunct to surgery. Neck skin differs from facial skin in thickness and dermal content. The goal of surgery is to reduce submental fullness and improve neck contour. Laser resurfacing of the neck simply improves the appearance of the skin. The laser should not be used to achieve significant additional tightening. These types of aggressive resurfacing procedures with high-density and deep penetration into the reticular dermis are more likely to result in significant complications (**Fig. 11**). The risk of laser-induced complications when treating the neck is reduced by lowering treatment density to approximately 50%, limiting ablation to the outer two-thirds of the epidermis, and even treating the upper and lower neck differently. The upper cervical skin above the first cervical rhytid resembles facial skin and thus can be treated similarly to undermined facial skin. However, the lower two-thirds

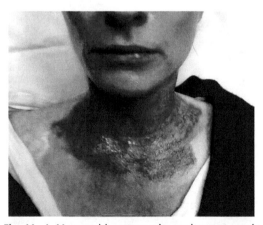

Fig. 11. A 44-year-old woman who underwent overly aggressive resurfacing of the neck. Although the density was only 30%, penetration into the reticular dermis was deep at 900 μm, resulting in second-degree burns. For this reason the author does not recommend deep fractional resurfacing of the face and neck after face and necklift surgery, respectively.

of the neck is significantly thinner with less skin adnexal appendages required for proper healing.

The Perioral Area

A facelift does little to improve perioral wrinkles. The author originally began to treat this area with a combination of deep fractional resurfacing at 450 μm and 15% to 20% density and single-pass fully ablative resurfacing at 100 μm. Although improvement was noticeable, patients were not satisfied because they had achieved greater improvements on other facial areas. This led to the author's decision 1 year ago to use more aggressive treatment parameters to treat deep perioral rhytids. At the time of this writing the author treats deep perioral rhytids by removing approximately 180 μm of epidermis and dermis. Results at this depth are comparable with those obtained with deep phenol peels, although healing times are 3 to 5 days longer than expected with single-pass ablative resurfacing (**Fig. 12**). Video 3 shows resurfacing of deep perioral rhytids.

For the nonfacelift patient, the combination of deep fractional and fully ablative CO_2 resurfacing can provide significant improvement in the face. Epidermal ablation, or superficial laser skin rejuvenation, is routinely used in combination with moderately deep dermal ablation to improve not only appearance of rhytids, but also to improve tightening by volumetric reduction. The large spot size (1–1.3 mm) removes most or all of the epidermis and the deeper fractional resurfacing removes "tissue volume."

Lower facial laxity can be improved to a modest degree with combination therapy. For the fractional modality, the author achieves modest tightening by treating to a depth of 500 to 600 μm with 20% to 30% density. Fully ablative laser treatment (100% density) is performed at 120 μm (**Fig. 13**).

Acne Scars

In the author's experience, laser resurfacing with either fully ablative or fractional CO_2 lasers alone produces only mild to moderate improvement in acne scars with any single treatment session. Although more favorable outcomes are obtained with multiple sessions, outcomes are optimized in a single session that includes fat grafting, subcision, and CO_2 laser resurfacing.

Combined laser therapies have been advocated to improve outcomes in acne scars.[34,35] The author has found that subcision is the key step to releasing scars. Subcision can be performed with a large needle, scissors, or a forked lipocannula. Tethered scars must be completely freed from underlying structures before treatment. If icepick

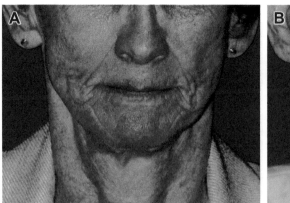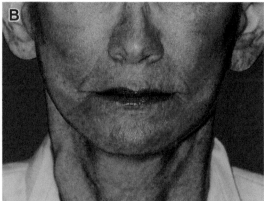

Fig. 12. A 67-year-old woman before (*A*) and after (*B*) treatment of deep perioral rhytids with a combination of deep fractional and fully ablative CO$_2$ laser procedures.

scars are present they may require vertical treatment with an 18-gauge needle or a laser beam of 1-mm spot size. A third choice is chemical reconstruction of skin scars.[36]

The cheek can be accessed from the hairline and widely undermined with scissors. The author prefers to have subcutaneous bridges in place because this may facilitate survival of fat which, when used, acts as a spacer to prevent scars

from retethering. Fat may be easily harvested from the abdomen or thigh under tumescent anesthesia. The author typically injects twice the desired amount of fat because of the lack of survivability of all the transferred fat. An added benefit of fat may include stem cell skin rejuvenation.

The author performs deep and superficial resurfacing for acne scars. Deep resurfacing should include a portion of the reticular dermis, which

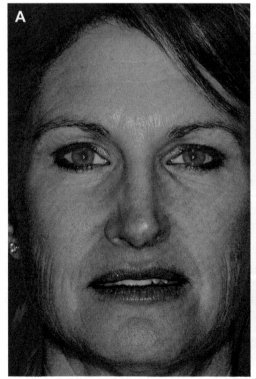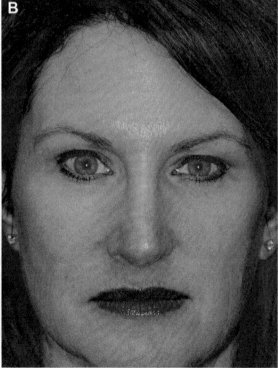

Fig. 13. A 46-year-old woman before (*A*) and after (*B*) treatment with a combination of fractional and fully ablative CO$_2$ laser procedures.

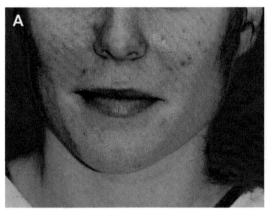 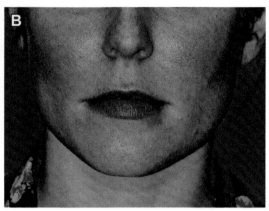

Fig. 14. A 27-year-old woman with acne scars before (*A*) treatment and after (*B*) subcision, fat grafting, and an aggressive fully ablative CO_2 laser procedure.

can be removed by treating to 800 μm depth and 20% to 30% density. Aggressive resurfacing to a depth of at least 200 μm with 100% density (fully ablative) removes all of epidermis and some papillary dermis resulting in better acne scar improvement. A clinical example is shown in **Fig. 14.**

SUMMARY

The concepts of fractional and fully ablative skin resurfacing will be discussed for many years. Although the novel idea of creating small microzones of ablation was revolutionary, the outcomes in the author's opinion were not. The results of fractional resurfacing simply did not produce the kind of results physicians and patients were expecting with a single treatment. Albeit great results with multiple fractional treatments can be achieved, none of these results matched those of well-performed single-treatment fully ablative treatments. By understanding the physics of skin ablation and then minimizing intraoperative and postoperative errors, consistent results with fully ablative treatments are achievable, which typically manage or exceed patient expectations.

SUPPLEMENTARY DATA

Supplementary data related to this article can be found online at http://dx.doi.org/10.1016/j.fsc. 2013.02.006.

REFERENCES

1. Manuskiatti W, Fitzpatrick RE, Goldman MP. Long-term effectiveness and side effects of carbon dioxide laser resurfacing for photoaged facial skin. J Am Acad Dermatol 1999;40:401–11.

2. Bernstein LJ, Kauvar AN, Grossman MC, et al. The short- and long-term side effects of carbon dioxide laser resurfacing. Dermatol Surg 1997;23:519–25.

3. Tierney EP, Eisen RF, Hanke CW. Fractionated CO2 laser skin rejuvenation. Dermatol Ther 2011; 24:41–53.

4. Shamsaldeen O, Peterson JD, Goldman MP. The adverse events of deep fractional CO(2): a retrospective study of 490 treatments in 374 patients. Lasers Surg Med 2011;43:453–6.

5. Alora MB, Anderson RR. Recent developments in cutaneous lasers. Lasers Surg Med 2000;26: 108–18.

6. Anderson RR. Laser-tissue interactions. In: Goldman MP, editor. Cutaneous laser surgery. 2nd edition. St Louis (MO): Mosby; 1999. p. 1–18.

7. Ross EV, McKinlay JR, Anderson RR. Why does carbon dioxide resurfacing work? A review. Arch Dermatol 1999;135:444–54.

8. Walsh JT Jr, Flotte TJ, Anderson RR, et al. Pulsed CO2 laser tissue ablation: effect of tissue type and pulse duration on thermal damage. Lasers Surg Med 1988;8:108–18.

9. Anderson RR, Parrish JA. Selective photothermolysis: precise microsurgery by selective absorption of pulsed radiation. Science 1983;220(4596):524–7.

10. Geronemus RG. Fractional photothermolysis: current and future applications. Lasers Surg Med 2006;38:169–76.

11. Kauvar AN. Laser skin resurfacing: perspectives at the millennium. Dermatol Surg 2000;26:174–7.

12. Kauvar AN, Waldorf HA, Geronemus RG. A histopathological comparison of "char-free" carbon dioxide lasers. Dermatol Surg 1996;22:343–8.

13. Choi B, Welch AJ. Analysis of thermal relaxation during laser irradiation of tissue. Lasers Surg Med 2001;29:351–9.

14. Khatri KA, Ross V, Grevelink JM, et al. Comparison of erbium:YAG and carbon dioxide lasers in

resurfacing of facial rhytides. Arch Dermatol 1999; 135:391–7.

15. Manstein D, Herron GS, Sink RK, et al. Fractional photothermolysis: a new concept for cutaneous remodeling using microscopic patterns of thermal injury. Lasers Surg Med 2004;34:426–38.

16. Ross EV, McKinlay JR, Sajben FP, et al. Use of a novel erbium laser in a Yucatan minipig: a study of residual thermal damage, ablation, and wound healing as a function of pulse duration. Lasers Surg Med 2002;30:93–100.

17. Nanni CA, Alster TS. Complications of carbon dioxide laser resurfacing. An evaluation of 500 patients. Dermatol Surg 1998;24:315–20.

18. Sriprachya-Anunt S, Fitzpatrick RE, Goldman MP, et al. Infections complicating pulsed carbon dioxide laser resurfacing for photoaged facial skin. Dermatol Surg 1997;23:527–35 [discussion: 535–6].

19. Schwartz RJ, Burns AJ, Rohrich RJ, et al. Long-term assessment of CO2 facial laser resurfacing: aesthetic results and complications. Plast Reconstr Surg 1999;103:592–601.

20. Berwald C, Levy JL, Magalon G. Complications of the resurfacing laser: retrospective study of 749 patients. Ann Chir Plast Esthet 2004;49:360–5.

21. Campbell TM, Goldman MP. Adverse events of fractionated carbon dioxide laser: review of 373 treatments. Dermatol Surg 2010;36:1645–50.

22. Khan MH, Sink RK, Manstein D, et al. Intradermally focused infrared laser pulses: thermal effects at defined tissue depths. Lasers Surg Med 2005;36: 270–80.

23. Grema H, Greve B, Raulin C. Facial rhytides: subsurfacing or resurfacing? A review. Lasers Surg Med 2003;32:405–12.

24. Hantash BM, Bedi VP, Kapadia B, et al. In vivo histological evaluation of a novel ablative fractional resurfacing device. Lasers Surg Med 2007; 39:96–107.

25. Reilly MJ, Cohen M, Hokugo A, et al. Molecular effects of fractional carbon dioxide laser resurfacing on photodamaged human skin. Arch Facial Plast Surg 2010;12:321–5.

26. Orringer JS, Kang S, Johnson TM, et al. Connective tissue remodeling induced by carbon dioxide laser resurfacing of photodamaged human skin. Arch Dermatol 2004;140:1326–32.

27. Berlin AL, Hussain M, Phelps R, et al. A prospective study of fractional scanned nonsequential carbon dioxide laser resurfacing: a clinical and histopathologic evaluation. Dermatol Surg 2009;35:222–8.

28. Tan KL, Kurniawati C, Gold MH. Low risk of postinflammatory hyperpigmentation in skin types 4 and 5 after treatment with fractional CO2 laser device. J Drugs Dermatol 2008;7:774–7.

29. Avram MM, Tope WD, Yu T, et al. Hypertrophic scarring of the neck following ablative fractional carbon dioxide laser resurfacing [Erratum appears in: Lasers Surg Med 2009;41:398]. Lasers Surg Med 2009;41:185–8.

30. Graber EM, Tanzi EL, Alster TS. Side effects and complications of fractional laser photothermolysis: experience with 961 treatments. Dermatol Surg 2008;34:301–5 [discussion: 305–7].

31. Ratner D, Tse Y, Marchell N, et al. Cutaneous laser resurfacing. J Am Acad Dermatol 1999;41(3 Pt 1): 365–89.

32. Davis SC, Cazzaniga AL, Ricotti C, et al. Topical oxygen emulsion. A novel wound therapy. Arch Dermatol 2007;143:1252–6.

33. Fife DJ, Fitzpatrick RE, Zachary CB. Complications of fractional CO2 laser resurfacing: four cases. Lasers Surg Med 2009;41:179–84.

34. Gentile RD. Combined laser treatment of actinic sun damage and acne scarring. Facial Plast Surg Clin North Am 2012;20:187–200, vi.

35. Rostan EF. Combining laser therapies for optimal outcomes in treating the aging face and acne scars. Facial Plast Surg Clin North Am 2012;20:221–9, vii.

36. Kim HJ, Kim TG, Kwon YS, et al. Comparison of a 1,550 nm Erbium: glass fractional laser and a chemical reconstruction of skin scars (CROSS) method in the treatment of acne scars: a simultaneous split-face trial. Lasers Surg Med 2009;41: 545–9.

Midface Injectable Fillers
Have They Replaced Midface Surgery?

Allison T. Pontius, MD[a],*, Scott R. Chaiet, MD[a,b],
Edwin F. Williams III, MD[a,b]

KEYWORDS

- Midface lift • Midface aging • Facial analysis • Midface fillers • Tear trough fillers
- Filler complications

KEY POINTS

- The understanding of midface aging has evolved in recent years with an emphasis on anatomically revolumizing the face over suspension alone.
- The fat of the midface is highly compartmentalized into deep and superficial compartments which lose volume and redistribute in an inferior direction with age.
- Injectable fillers offer a versatile, safe, and effective means to create an aesthetically pleasing midface/periorbital complex.
- Both surgical midface lifting with fat transfer and injectable fillers to the midface share the common goal of creating a youthful eyelid/cheek contour.

 A video demonstrating injection of a patient with calcium hydroxylapatite in the midface and with hyaluronic acid in the tear trough can be viewed online at http://www.facialplastic.theclinics.com/

OVERVIEW

Since 1995, the senior author (E.F.W.) has been a strong proponent of midface lifting using an extended minimal incision approach suspending the entire midface as a single anatomic unit.[1–9] Approximately 1200 procedures have been performed over this 15-year period. Beginning in 2004, the senior author began incorporating fat transfer as a complementary component to the midface lift,[4] and currently performs fat transfer in 95% of all midface lifting procedures. The use of fat transfer in conjunction with the midface lift is to augment midface volume and address hollowness in the tear trough/infraorbital complex, which creates a more aesthetically pleasing result than midface lifting alone. Although this remains an effective and reliable procedure, we have seen a significant shift in our practice to less-invasive treatments for the midface and tear trough. The understanding of the pathophysiology of midface aging has evolved in recent years with an emphasis on anatomically revolumizing the face over suspension alone. We have found that, in most patients, injectable fillers offer a versatile, safe, and effective means to create an aesthetically pleasing midface/periorbital complex. The injectable fillers are appealing for patients because

Disclosures/Conflict of Interest: E.F. Williams, III, MD, FACS is a shareholder of Allergan stock and has previously been a principal investigator for clinical trials for Allergan and Sanofi-Aventis. A.T. Pontius, MD and S.R. Chaiet, MD: None.
[a] Facial Plastic and Reconstructive Surgery, Williams' Center of Plastic Surgery Specialists, 1072 Troy Schenectady Road, Latham, NY 12110, USA; [b] Division of Otolaryngology-Head and Neck Surgery, Department of Surgery, Albany Medical Center, 47 New Scotland Avenue, Albany, NY 12208, USA
* Corresponding author.
E-mail address: allisonpontius@ymail.com

Facial Plast Surg Clin N Am 21 (2013) 229–239
http://dx.doi.org/10.1016/j.fsc.2013.02.012

of less downtime and less cost than traditional surgery. Particularly with a younger patient population seeking midface/periorbital rejuvenation, injectable fillers are a viable option for these patients who neither need nor want a surgical procedure.

In this article, we explore the reasons for the increasing use of less-invasive procedures for midface rejuvenation and how fillers are changing traditional approaches to the midface.

VOLUME CHANGES IN THE AGING MIDFACE

The fat of the midface is compartmentalized into a deep and a superficial layer. The deep layer is composed of the deep cheek fat and the sub-orbicularis oculi fat.[10] The superficial layer, or "malar fat,"[11] is composed of 3 fat compartments: the nasolabial, superior medial cheek, and inferior infraorbital fat (**Fig. 1**). The aging midface experiences volume loss not only of the deep and superficial fat compartments but also in other components of the face, including skin, muscle, and bone. In a study of computed tomography scans, Shaw and colleagues[12] demonstrated that the bony structures of the orbit undergo morphologic change with a widening of the orbital aperture that likely contributes to the change in the appearance of the overlying soft tissue envelope of the aging periorbital complex. They also found that the maxillary angle significantly decreased with age. The decrease in maxillary angle may lead to decreased skeletal support for the malar fat pad, which may allow the nasolabial crease to become more prominent with age. In another

study of computed tomography scans, the midface fat compartments were analyzed for aging changes.[13] The study further clarified facial fat anatomy and developed concepts of age-dependant changes in midfacial fat compartments: an inferior migration of the fat compartments and an inferior volume shift within the compartments in addition to volume loss. The investigators found that the inferior migration of midface fat compartments is due not only to gravity but is also a consequence of volume loss of the buccal extension of the buccal fat pad.[13] A deflation of this fat compartment will lead to lack of support of the medial cheek and the middle cheek fat. Additionally, the fat within each compartment was found to redistribute in an inferior direction. Therefore, as we plan our rejuvenation of the midface (either surgically or with fillers) we must consider both soft tissue volume loss and bony loss.

TREATMENT GOALS

Both surgical midface lifting with fat transfer and injectable fillers to the midface share the common goal of creating a youthful eyelid/cheek contour. When deciding which approach to use, we consider the following factors (**Fig. 2**):

- Severity of soft tissue ptosis
- Degree of volume loss
- Presence of significant brow ptosis
- Patient age
- Patient willingness for downtime
- Cost

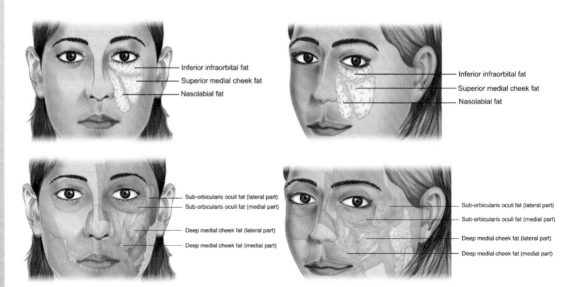

Fig. 1. Diagram of deep and superficial fat compartments of the midface.

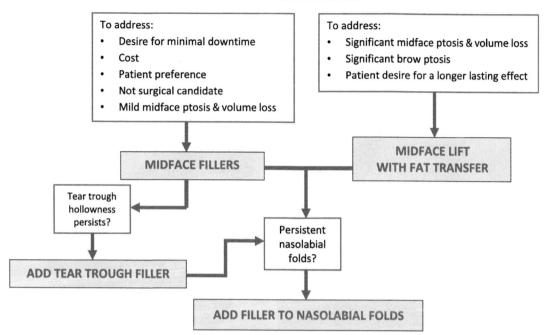

MIDFACE VOLUME LOSS

To address:
- Desire for minimal downtime
- Cost
- Patient preference
- Not surgical candidate
- Mild midface ptosis & volume loss

To address:
- Significant midface ptosis & volume loss
- Significant brow ptosis
- Patient desire for a longer lasting effect

MIDFACE FILLERS

MIDFACE LIFT WITH FAT TRANSFER

Tear trough hollowness persists?

Persistent nasolabial folds?

ADD TEAR TROUGH FILLER

ADD FILLER TO NASOLABIAL FOLDS

Fig. 2. Decision algorithm for determining injectable fillers to the midface versus surgical midface lifting with fat transfer.

- Patient preference
- Patient's surgical candidacy

PATIENT SELECTION

Most patients are viable candidates for injectable fillers. The patients for whom surgery is encouraged are those

- With significant midface and brow ptosis (our technique for midface lifting is done in conjunction with a browlift[6,8])
- With extensive facial volume loss who would benefit more from panfacial fat transfer
- Who desire a longer-lasting result

The remainder of patients are candidates for filler injection, although the ideal patient would be young (in their 40s) with good skin tone with mild-moderate midface volume loss, tear trough deformity, and nasolabial folds (**Fig. 3** and Video demonstrating midface and tear trough injection).

PRETREATMENT PLANNING

Planning begins with a thorough facial analysis.

When considering the midface, we first evaluate its bony structure. The malar eminence (the most prominent portion of the zygomatic bone) is identified and palpated. The location of the malar eminence may not be prominent or symmetric on both sides of the face. It is often helpful to mark out the location of the malar region using a standard technique, such as the Hinderer method.[14]

Mark the Malar Region

The Hinderer method helps locate the malar eminence at a point of intersection of 2 lines. The first line connects the nasal ala to the tragus and the second line connects the commissure of the lip to the lateral canthus (**Fig. 4**). The area posterior and superior to the crossing of Hinderer lines is the most prominent part of the midface, and where the lines intersect usually identifies the area of maximal malar flattening.[14,15] We find it helpful to mark these areas out on the patient's face before injection. Once the malar eminence and the area of maximal malar flattening are identified, then the region for injection is marked out in a "triangular" shape (**Fig. 5**).

1. The apex of the triangle is at the malar eminence
2. The corner of the upside-down triangle is superomedial (just inferior to the infraorbital rim)
3. The third point is just superior to the middle of the nasolabial fold

By using a combination of direct palpation of the soft tissue and bony constituents of the malar

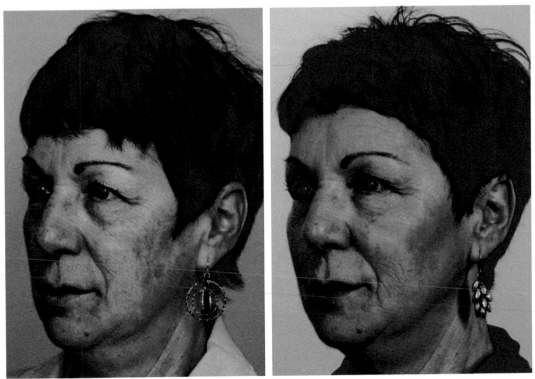

Fig. 3. Oblique photograph of a patient 2 weeks after receiving calcium hydroxylapatite midface injection (1.5 mL per side) with hyaluronic acid tear trough injection (0.5 mL per side). She is an ideal candidate for a surgical midface/brow lift (with blepharoplasty), but the patient preferred nonsurgical treatment. Subtle tear trough injection was performed to avoid emphasizing the underlying dermatochalasis. Video of this patient's injection can be seen in the online version of this article at http://www.facialplastic.theclinics.com/.

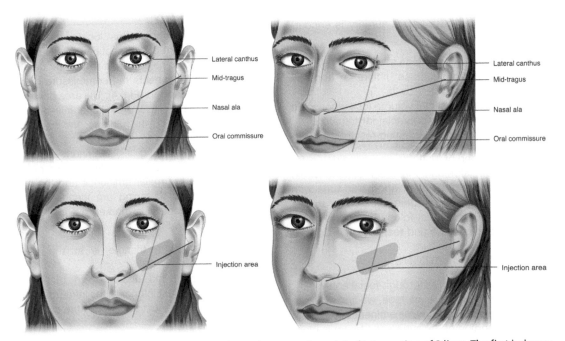

Fig. 4. The Hinderer method to locate the malar eminence at the point of intersection of 2 lines. The first is drawn from the nasal ala to tragus and the second line connects the commissure of the lip to lateral canthus.

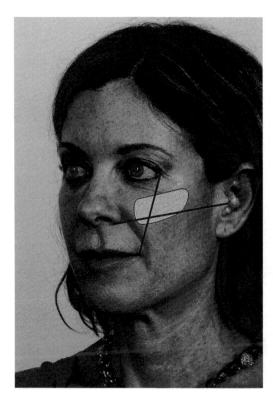

Fig. 5. Patient with Hinderer lines drawn and the area marked out in the midface for injectable filler.

eminence and marking out Hinderer lines, the areas for injection are delineated.

Assess Ptosis and Volume Loss

Next, the degree of ptosis and volume loss in the deep and superficial fat compartments of the face are assessed to determine how much filler will be needed. The deep medial fat is important to augment to increase anterior projection, improve the tear trough, and diminish the nasolabial fold.[16]

Choice of Filler

We typically perform this with a thicker filler, such as calcium hydroxylapatite (Radiesse; Merz/Bioform, San Mateo, CA). However, other choices include poly-L-lactic acid (Sculptra; Sanofi-Aventis U.S. LLC, Bridgewater, NJ), which is a collagen stimulator as opposed to a filler. Poly-L-lactic acid's effects are usually subtler than calcium hydroxylapatite (Radiesse, Merz/Bioform) and multiple treatment sessions are required to achieve a comparable effect. However, the duration of poly-L-lactic acid (Sculptra, Sanofi-Aventis U.S. LLC) is longer than most fillers, lasting up to 2 years. Another option is a hyaluronic acid filler, such as Juvederm Ultra Plus (Allergan Inc, Irvine, CA) or Perlane (Medicis, Scottsdale, AZ). We usually use hyaluronic acid fillers for more superficial injections or fine-tuning after a deeper injection has been performed. When using hyaluronic acid fillers in a deeper plane, we have found that a greater volume of product is necessary to achieve an effect comparable to a more substantial filler like calcium hydroxylapatite (Radiesse, Merz/Bioform). In general, hyaluronic acid fillers are the best choice for injecting in the subdermal plane; however, we do feel that primary correction of significant midface volume loss should not focus on the superficial layer alone. If excess hyaluronic acid is placed subdermally in the midface, it tends to give the face a doughy appearance with an unnaturally thick superficial layer.

Assess Tear Troughs and Midface as Single Unit

After injection of the midface, the tear troughs are again assessed. It is important to consider the midface and tear troughs as a single unit. To address one without consideration of the other will usually lead to a less then optimal result. The tear troughs may be significantly corrected following midface injection, particularly if the deep medial fat was injected (**Fig. 6**). Deep midface injections tend to shift the shadow of the hollowed infraorbital rim in an upward direction, which effectively shortens the length of the lower lid and improves its appearance. If the tear troughs remain hollowed after midface injection, then they may be filled judiciously with a hyaluronic acid filler (Restylane, Medicis).

Assess Nasolabial Folds

Finally, improvement in the nasolabial fold is examined after the midface augmentation is performed and then, if indicated, a small amount of hyaluronic acid filler (Juvederm Ultra Plus, Allergan Inc, or Perlane, Medicis) can be injected to further efface the nasolabial folds.

PREPARATION
Medications

Before the scheduled injection, the patient should have a thorough consultation to discuss any medical conditions, medications (including supplements), allergies, bleeding tendencies, and any previous cosmetic procedures (injections or surgery) to the face. Patients should be advised to discontinue medications that may cause bleeding (eg, aspirin, nonsteroidal anti-inflammatory agents) and supplements (eg, fish oil, green tea, garlic, ginseng, vitamin E) 7 to 10 days before treatment.

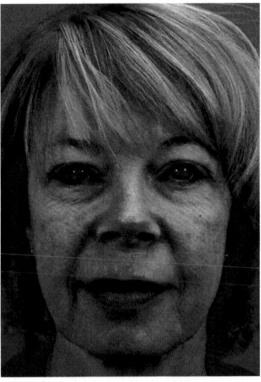 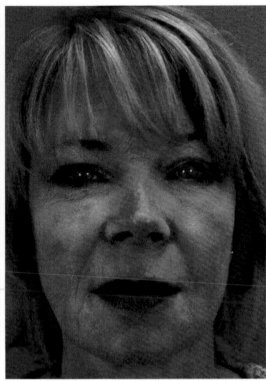

Fig. 6. Before and after photographs of patient with calcium hydroxylapatite injection to the midface. Note the improvement in the tear troughs. Hyaluronic acid injection was not needed after midface injection.

If the patient is on a blood-thinning medication (aspirin, nonsteroidal anti-inflammatory agents, warfarin [Coumadin; Bristol-Myers Squibb Pharma, Bridgewater, NJ] or clopidogrel bisulfate [Plavix; Sanofi-Aventis]) for a medical condition in which the risk of stopping the medication may outweigh the benefits, then it is recommended to continue anticoagulation for minor dermatologic procedures with low risk of bleeding.[17] However, whether one chooses to proceed with injections should be based on the practitioner's best medical judgment and should be deferred if it is deemed unsafe.

Preoperative Photos

In preparation for midface and tear trough injections, the patient should have standard aesthetic photographic views taken (frontal, lateral, and oblique). These should be displayed on a monitor in the injection room or printed and hung on the wall for reference during the injection.

Face Cleanse

The patient is asked to cleanse the face to remove all make-up before injection.

PROCEDURE SET-UP
Midface Injection

For the midface injection, one will need a Mayo stand set-up with the following items:

- Alcohol swabs to cleanse the skin
- A marker (we use a white eyeliner pencil)
- An ice pack
- 1% lidocaine with 1:100,000 epinephrine in a 1-mL syringe with a 30-gauge needle
- A female-to-female luer lock connector and two 3.0-mL mixing syringes
- Several 4 × 4 gauze sponges
- Two 27-gauge 1.5-inch needles
- The calcium hydroxylapatite (Radiesse, Merz/Bioform)

Typically we use the 1.5-mL volume of calcium hydroxylapatite (Radiesse, Merz/Bioform) per side, although the amount of product for any individual patient may vary.

Tear Trough Injection

For the tear trough set-up, the Mayo stand holds the following:

- Alcohol swabs
- A skin marker (white eyeliner)

- 1% lidocaine with 1:100,000 epinephrine in a 1-mL syringe with a 30-gauge needle
- A 27-gauge × 1.5-inch blunt cannula (Dermasculpt, CosmoFrance, Inc, Miami Beach, FL)
- One 25-gauge 0.5-inch needle
- An ice pack
- A 1-mL syringe of hyaluronic acid (Restylane, Medicis)

PROCEDURAL APPROACH/TECHNIQUE
Midface Injection

- The patient is evaluated sitting in an upright position. Once the area of maximum volume loss has been defined by a combination of visualization, palpation, and Hinderer lines, the area of injection is marked out in a triangular shape, as described previously. The patient is reclined approximately 30° to facilitate injection. We prefer calcium hydroxylapatite (Radiesse, Merz/Bioform) for correction in this area.
- Before injection, the calcium hydroxylapatite (Radiesse, Merz/Bioform) is diluted with 0.5 to 1.0 mL of 1% plain lidocaine (per 1.5-mL syringe of calcium hydroxylapatite [Radiesse, Merz/Bioform]).

Note: Admixing lidocaine into calcium hydroxylapatite at treatment is approved by the Food and Drug Administration and is described on the package insert. This gives a thinner consistency to the product and facilitates placement while providing the patient with local anesthesia.

- Additional anesthesia consists only of approximately 0.2 mL of 1% lidocaine with 1:100,000 epinephrine at the needle insertion sites.
- The filler is placed in a cross-hatching fashion from 2 injection sites, with the area of maximal cross hatching corresponding to the area of maximal malar flattening.
- The first site is the inferomedial point of the triangle and the second site is superolateral near the malar eminence.
- The product is placed slowly in a retrograde manner.
- It is placed in a deep tissue plane in the area of maximal volume loss and then slightly less product is tapered laterally toward the malar eminence to create a pleasing contour rather than remaining centered only on the deep medial fat pad. This helps to recreate the inverted triangular shape of a youthful face (**Fig. 7**).

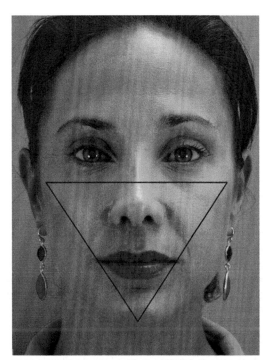

Fig. 7. Illustration with inverted triangle overlay on a youthful face.

Tear Trough Injection

- The tear trough is treated with a hyaluronic acid gel filler (Restylane, Medicis) using a flexible 25-gauge × 1.5-inch blunt cannula (Dermasculpt, CosmoFrance, Inc).
- The true tear trough is injected first and the lateral portion of the infraorbital rim second (if needed).
- The cannula entry point is marked inferior and lateral to the plane of the tear trough.
- Approximately 0.1 mL of 1% lidocaine with 1:100,000 epinephrine is injected at this site. No further anesthesia is necessary.
- Using a 27-gauge 0.5-inch needle, a small puncture is made in the skin. The cannula is inserted through this puncture and advanced toward the medial canthus, ensuring the depth of the cannula is below the orbicularis oculi muscle.
- Slowly, the product is placed in a retrograde fashion in linear threads. This is performed several times until improvement in the tear trough is noted.
- If the patient also has hollowness in the lateral portion of the infraorbital rim, further injection can be performed laterally. Using the same insertion site, the 27-gauge needle is used again to facilitate entry of the cannula; however, this time the cannula is directed superolateral.

Note: It can be more difficult to advance the cannula in this direction, because mild pressure is needed to break through small fibrous attachments.

- The total amount of product injected is rarely more than 1.0 mL per side.
- After injection is complete, a small amount of molding is done with the fingertips to smooth out any irregularities.

POTENTIAL COMPLICATIONS AND THEIR MANAGEMENT
Common Complications

The most common complications of injectable fillers are injection site erythema, swelling, pain, and bruising. These usually last for a few days and resolve uneventfully. These early complications can be minimized by the use of ice or cold compresses immediately after the injection.

Serious Complications/Events

More serious adverse events include allergic reactions, infections, vascular compromise, and placement of product that is too superficial.[18] True hypersensitivity reactions to hyaluronic acid fillers are rare, occurring in 1 in 5000 cases.[19] Infection is also uncommon and can be managed with antibiotics or antivirals, depending on clinical features. Injection in the perioral area can reactive herpes simplex virus and patients prone to cold sores are treated prophylactically with antivirals.

Tissue Necrosis

The most potentially serious complication is tissue necrosis caused by interruption of the vascular supply to an area by direct injury of the vessel, compression of the area surrounding the vessel, or obstruction of the vessel with filler material. The first sign of injection necrosis is painless blanching or bruising of the immediate area of injection.[20] This usually occurs immediately at the time of injection but has been reported up to 6 hours later.[21] A protocol for treatment has been described by Glaich and colleagues.[20] If a significant area of blanching occurs while injecting, immediately discontinue the injection and gently massage the treated area. To encourage vasodilatation, place a gauze soaked in warm water on the area. Nitroglycerin paste is then used for more significant vasodilation. If signs of impending injection necrosis following injection of a hyaluronic acid filler occur, hyaluronidase can be used to decompress occluded vessels. It is important for anyone performing filler injections to have a detailed emergency protocol easily accessible and to have nitroglycerin paste and hyaluronidase readily available.

Visible Lumps and Tyndall Effect

Too superficial placement of filler may lead to immediate lumps or bumps and can be avoided by appropriate technique and gentle product massage after injection. Additionally, superficial placement of hyaluronic acid fillers in the dermis can result in the Tyndall effect, particularly in the periorbital area. The Tyndall effect is a blue discoloration caused by the refraction of light from the clear gel visible superficially in the skin.[19] The Tyndall effect can be avoided when injecting a tear trough deformity by placement of the filler below the orbicularis oculi muscle.[22] Also, care should be taken with injecting calcium hydroxylapatite near the infraorbital nerve. Cases of prolonged anesthesia and paresthesia in the distribution of the infraorbital nerve have been reported.[19]

Late Complications

Late complications include migration, discoloration, scarring, atrophy, and foreign body granulomas.[18] Causes of granulomas include the volume of injected material, size of the filler particles used, impurities, and biofilms.[23] Granulomas can effectively be treated with steroid injection.[24]

IMMEDIATE POSTINJECTION CARE

Immediately following injection, the patient is reclined in the chair and given a cold compress to hold over the treated areas for 10 minutes to minimize swelling and ecchymoses. Patients are told to avoid strenuous exercise for the remainder of the day and to sleep on their back with their head slightly elevated to avoid pressure on the treated areas. They may use ice or cold compresses off and on for the next 24 hours as needed.

RECOVERY

Patients typically have a brief recovery period after the procedure. The treated areas are often slightly erythematous for the remainder of the day. Patients may experience mild swelling of the midface and/or tear trough and this may persist for up to a week. We find that ecchymoses are uncommon, especially for the tear trough injection. We suggest a follow-up appointment 2 to 3 months after the initial injection to reassess the degree of augmentation following degradation of the gel carrier of the calcium hydroxylapatite (Radiesse, Merz/Bioform). However, as the gel is phagocytized, the process of neocollagenesis begins in and around the microspheres, stimulating the gradual growth of the patient's own collagen, which may obviate the need for touch-up injections at this time.[25] In our experience, both the midface and tear trough region maintain their result for approximately 1 year.

SUMMARY

Our understanding of the midface anatomy and its aging process continues to evolve. There is no single algorithm of treatment that will work for every patient. What we do know is that the fat of the midface is highly compartmentalized into deep and superficial compartments. The most recent computed tomography studies have even further defined the midface fat compartments into 2, and paranasally, 3 independent anatomic layers.[13] Additionally, we now understand that bony changes of the midface and orbit contribute to the aging process.[12] A lack of structural support provided by the midfacial bony structures combined with the deflation, inferior migration, and an inferior volume shift of fat within their compartments all are contributors to the midfacial aging process. Consequently, to thoroughly restore the youthful aesthetics of the midface we must restore these changes. These changes may also vary in degree from patient to patient. We believe there is no one way to correct these changes. For some patients, midface lifting with fat transfer is the answer and for other patients an optimal aesthetic outcome is created with strategically placed fillers (**Table 1**). We find more and more patients are opting for fillers usually because they are seeking a less-invasive way to treat the aging process. Also, the younger patients tend to opt for fillers because they want to delay surgery, want minimal downtime, and want to minimize the cost of treatment. Our approach with fillers is to create an aesthetically pleasing face. Simple volumization without an aesthetic eye or anatomic understanding does not create an attractive midface. An attractive adult midface does not have full "apple" cheeks but has clean, defined cheekbones and a subtle concavity below them. To create this

Table 1
Summary comparison of midface surgery versus midface injectable fillers

	Midface Surgery	Midface Injectable Fillers
Patient selection	Significant soft tissue and bony volume loss Severe soft tissue ptosis Presence of brow ptosis More significant cost but longer-lasting results	Less cost of traditional surgery Younger patient (40s) with good skin tone seeking rejuvenation who neither needs nor wants a surgical procedure Patient not surgical candidate
Preoperative planning	Determine degree of ptosis and volume loss in deep and superficial fat compartments Evaluate need for nasolabial fold effacement Identify donor site for lipotransfer	Determine degree of ptosis and volume loss in deep and superficial fat compartments Examine tear trough for hyaluronic acid filler need Evaluate need for nasolabial fold effacement
Preoperative preparation	Discontinue standard medications and supplements Standard aesthetic photography	Discontinue standard medications and supplements Standard aesthetic photography
Complications	For fat injection: Injection site erythema, swelling, pain, and bruising Injection of fat that is too superficial For midface surgery: Asymmetry, infection, hematoma, facial nerve neuropraxia, trigeminal nerve paraesthesia, alopecia and scarring	Injection site erythema, swelling, pain, and bruising Allergic reaction to product (rare) Infection Vascular compromise Placement of product that is too superficial (Late: migration, discoloration, scarring, atrophy, and foreign body granulomas)
Recovery	Approximately two weeks	Less downtime than traditional surgery Slight erythema on day of injection and mild swelling of the midface and/or tear trough for up to a week

shape, we use a calcium hydroxylapatite filler (Radiesse, Merz/Bioform) for injections into the deep fat and extend this injection to the malar eminence in a symmetric, triangular fashion. Rohrich and colleagues[16] found that injection into the deep medial fat compartment improved midface projection and recreated a youthful cheek, improved the V-deformity of the lower lid, and diminished the prominence of the nasolabial fold. We have found this to be the case as well. However, if a tear trough deformity persists after midface augmentation, then we recommend a tear trough injection with a hyaluronic acid filler (Restylane, Medicis) performed at the same time as midface augmentation or as a second procedure.

Finally, to answer the opening question on whether fillers have replaced the midface lift, our answer is both yes and no. Surgery may be the best approach for patients with significant midface soft tissue ptosis that would not be corrected with volume restoration alone. Additionally, if the patient has concurrent brow ptosis, we would guide the patient to a surgical treatment that restores both brow position and midface descent. Patient preference for a long-lasting result would also be a reason to undergo midface surgery. However, in the past few years, more and more of our patients select (and are guided to) nonsurgical injections, and we feel satisfied that we can deliver an aesthetically pleasing result using a combination of fillers with an anatomic approach to volumization.

SUPPLEMENTARY DATA

Supplementary data related to this article can be found online at http://dx.doi.org/10.1016/j.fsc.2013.02.012.

REFERENCES

1. DeFatta RJ, Williams EF 3rd. Midface lifting: current standards. Facial Plast Surg 2011;27(1):77–85.
2. Yeh CC, Williams EF 3rd. Midface restoration in the management of the lower eyelid. Facial Plast Surg Clin North Am 2010;18(3):365–74.
3. DeFatta RJ, Williams EF 3rd. Evolution of midface rejuvenation. Arch Facial Plast Surg 2009;11(1):6–12.
4. Pontius AT, Williams EF 3rd. The evolution of midface rejuvenation: combining the midface lift and fat transfer. Arch Facial Plast Surg 2006;8(5):300–5.
5. Krishna S, Williams EF 3rd. Lipocontouring in conjunction with the minimal incision brow and subperiosteal midface lift: the next dimension in midface rejuvenation. Facial Plast Surg Clin North Am 2006; 14(3):221–8.
6. Pontius AT, Williams EF 3rd. The extended minimal incision approach to midface rejuvenation. Facial Plast Surg Clin North Am 2005;13(3):411–9.
7. Batniji RK, Williams EF. Effects of subperiosteal midfacial elevation via an endoscopic brow-lift incision on lower facial rejuvenation. Facial Plast Surg 2005;21(1):33–7.
8. Lam SM, Chang EW, Rhee JS, et al. Perspective: rejuvenation of the periocular region: a unified approach to the eyebrow, midface and eyelid complex. Ophthal Plast Reconstr Surg 2004;20(1):1–9.
9. Williams EF 3rd, Vargas H, Dahiya R, et al. Midfacial rejuvenation via a minimal-incision brow-lift approach: critical evaluation of a 5-year experience. Arch Facial Plast Surg 2003;5(6):470–8.
10. Rohrich RJ, Arbique GM, Wong C, et al. The anatomy of the suborbicularis fat: implications for periorbirtal rejuvenation. Plast Reconstr Surg 2008; 124:946–51.
11. Owsley JQ. Lifting the malar fat pad for correction of prominent nasolabial folds. Plast Reconstr Surg 1993;91:463–74 [discussion: 475–6].
12. Shaw RB, Katzel EB, Koltz PF, et al. Aging of the facial skeleton: aesthetic implications and rejuvenation strategies. Plast Reconstr Surg 2010;127: 374–83.
13. Gierloff M, Stohring C, Buder T, et al. Aging changes of the midfacial fat compartments: a computed tomographic study. Plast Reconstr Surg 2011;129: 263–73.
14. Nechala P, Mahoney J, Farkas LG. Comparison of techniques used to locate the malar eminence. Can J Plast Surg 2000;8(1):21–4.
15. Cattin TA. A single injection technique for midface rejuvenation. J Cosmet Dermatol 2010;9:256–9.
16. Rohrich RJ, Pessa JE, Ristow B. The youthful cheek and the deep medial fat compartment. Plast Reconstr Surg 2008;121:2107–12.
17. Douketis JD, Berger PB, Dunn AS, et al. The perioperative management of antithrombotic therapy: American College of Chest Physicians Evidence-Based Clinical Practice Guidelines (8th edition). Chest 2008;133(Suppl):299S–339S.
18. Nguyen AT, Ahmad J, Fagien S, et al. Cosmetic medicine: facial resurfacing and injectables. Plast Reconstr Surg 2012;129:142e–53e.
19. Jones D. Volumizing the face with soft tissue fillers. Clin Plast Surg 2011;38:379–90.
20. Glaich AS, Cohen JL, Goldberg LH. Injection necrosis of the glabella: protocol for prevention and treatment after use of dermal fillers. Dermatol Surg 2006;32:276–81.
21. Hirsch RJ, Cohen JL, Carruthers JD. Successful management of an unusual presentation of impending necrosis following a hyaluronic acid injection embolus and a proposed algorithm for management with hyaluronidase. Dermatol Surg 2007;33:357–60.

22. Hirsch RJ, Carruthers JD, Carruthers A. Infraorbitral hollow treatment by dermal fillers. Dermatol Surg 2007;33:1116–9.

23. Lemperle G, Gauthier-Hazan N, Wolters M, et al. Foreign body granulomas after all injectable dermal fillers: part 1. Possible causes. Plast Reconstr Surg 2009;123:1842–63.

24. Lemperle G, Gauthier-Hazan N. Foreign body granulomas after all injectable dermal fillers: part 2. Treatment options. Plast Reconstr Surg 2009;123:1864–73.

25. Coleman KM, Voights R, CeVore DP, et al. Neocollagenesis after injection of calcium hydroxylapatite composition in a canine model. Dermatol Surg 2008;34:S53–5.

Nonsurgical Rhinoplasty Using Dermal Fillers

Michael E. Jasin, MD

KEYWORDS

- Nonsurgical rhinoplasty • Dermal fillers • Calcium hydroxylapatite • Hyaluronic acid
- Correction of nasal defects • Injectables • Semipermanent duration

KEY POINTS

- Nonsurgical rhinoplasty can be appropriate for patients who are reluctant to undergo surgical intervention.
- Effects are long lasting but not permanent.
- Posttreatment downtime is minimal.
- Calcium hydroxylapatite is the dermal filler of choice for nonsurgical rhinoplasty, because of its duration, moldability, high viscosity, and elasticity.
- Hyaluronic acids with high viscosity and elasticity are acceptable alternatives.

INTRODUCTION

We are in the middle of a new era of rhinoplasty, in which surgery is not the only means to address nasal defects. Nonsurgical options seem more viable than they would have been before the advent of various synthetic injectable fillers. These fillers have greater longevity and rheological properties more conducive to facial contouring than earlier nonsurgical products. As a consequence, nonsurgical rhinoplasty is becoming increasingly more popular. Many patients are now choosing to bypass permanent surgical correction in favor of a noninvasive, albeit impermanent, method for nasal recontouring.

This article outlines the evolution of nonsurgical rhinoplasty and identifies properties to consider when selecting which dermal filler to use. It includes a description of the types of nasal deformities that can be treated with injectables, as well as the role of nonsurgical rhinoplasty in a comprehensive regimen for correction of nasal deformities.

THE EVOLUTION OF NONSURGICAL RHINOPLASTY

Initial reports of injectable contouring or nonsurgical rhinoplasty date back to the middle of the 1980s. At the time, treatment options were limited to bovine collagen and silicone. However, since that time, semipermanent dermal fillers have increasingly been noted in the literature as acceptable formulations for nonsurgical rhinoplasty. Although use of dermal fillers in nonsurgical rhinoplasty remains an off-label application of hyaluronic acids (HA) and calcium hydroxylapatite (CaHA), their use in correction of nasal deformities has been widely reported in the clinical literature over the years, as shown in **Table 1**.

SELECTING THE APPROPRIATE FILLER FOR NONSURGICAL RHINOPLASTY

The available choices of fillers for nonsurgical rhinoplasty primarily include cross-linked HA

Dr Jasin is a board-certified facial plastic surgeon in private practice on the Gulf Coast of Florida. Dr Jasin has received consulting fees for his work with Merz Aesthetics (San Mateo, CA), is a member of the Merz Aesthetics Advisory Board and Medical Education Faculty, and has held privately purchased stock in the corporation.
Jasin Facial Rejuvenation Institute, 13801 Bruce B. Downs Boulevard, Suite 305, Tampa, FL 33613, USA
E-mail address: mjasin@aol.com

Table 1
Clinical literature overview of use of dermal fillers in nonsurgical rhinoplasty

Reference	Filler/Procedure	Key Points of Study
Knapp and Vistnes,[1] 1985	Bovine collagen/surgical depressions resulting from rhinoplasty	Short-term filler may retain correction indefinitely
Webster et al,[2] 1986	Medical grade silicone/injected subdermally for postrhinoplasty defects	347 patients/1937 treatments; recommended undercorrection because filler stimulates indigenous collagen growth
Han et al,[3] 2006	Restylane (Q-Med, Uppsala, Sweden) coupled with autologous fibroblasts from harvested dermis/augmentation rhinoplasty	11 patients; 10%–40% resorption in the first 6 mo in 6 patients; stabilization at 6 mo. Minor surgery rather than noninvasive as a result of epidermal flap necessary for harvesting. Used fibroblasts to increase longevity
Beer,[4] 2006	Restylane/postrhinoplasty defect of nasal dorsum	Case report of 1 patient: safe, inexpensive, well-tolerated; mention of CaHA as alternative
Becker,[5] 2006	Radiesse (Merz Aesthetics, San Mateo, CA)/Nonsurgical rhinoplasty	25 patients, 15 with previous surgical rhinoplasty; viable alternative to surgery; preferred CaHA caused by moldability and durability; mean patient satisfaction 7.9/10
Rokhasar and Ciocon,[6] 2008	Radiesse/primary correction of nasal deformities	14 patients; no significant complications, high patient satisfaction
De Lacerda and Zancannaro,[7] 2007	Porcine collagens and HAs/filler rhinoplasty vs augmentation rhinoplasty	Filler rhinoplasty perhaps more accurate term than augmentation because of creating illusion of smaller nose through augmentation
Cassuto,[8] 2009	Evolence (Ortho Dermatologics, Skillman, NJ)/nonsurgical rhinoplasty	12 patients; mean follow-up of 8 mo with stable correction
Siclovan and Jomah,[9] 2009	Evolence/nasal deformities and postrhinoplasty irregularities	Correction for up to 1 y
Humphrey et al,[10] 2009	HAs, CaHA, silicone review article	HA/CaHA safest available agents for nasal dorsum and sidewall deformities. Caution against filler in tip of nose
Rivkin and Solieman-zadeh,[11] 2009	CaHA in nonsurgical rhinoplasty	4-y retrospective study of 385 patients (295 for follow-up). 46% required touch-up 2 mo after initial treatment; 28% touch-up 2–6 mo after initial treatment; 18% touch-up 6 mo to 1 y after initial treatment. AE: prolonged erythema (more prevalent in postsurgical rhinoplasty patients) with 2 cases of partial skin necrosis and 6 cases of cellulitis
Bray et al,[12] 2010	Restylane/nonsurgical nasal augmentation and postrhinoplasty asymmetry	Duration up to 18 mo; mention of CaHA to treat internal valve collapse
Dayan and Kempiners, 2005[13]	Botulinum toxin either alone or with injectable fillers/nasal tip ptosis and acute nasolabial angle	5 units of botulinum toxin in depressor septi muscle bilaterally and 3 units into each levator labii superioris alaeque nasi muscle
Monreal,[14] 2011	Autologous fat transfer/stand-alone correction or with surgical rhinoplasty	33 patients, 36 treatments; grafting to radix, glabella, pyriform aperture. Volume decrease first 15–30 d, stable thereafter. Duration unknown
Kim and Ahn,[15] 2012	Radiesse/nonsurgical augmentation in Asian population	87 patients, 4 complications: 1 dorsal asymmetry (corrected), 1 overinjection of columella-labial angle causing intraoral submucosal nodule, 1 self-limited dermatitis, 1 inflammation/erythema at injection site; plane was subdermal with CaHA and intradermal with HA for tip

products (Restylane [Medicis Aesthetics, Scottsdale, AZ], Perlane [Medicis Aesthetics, Scottsdale, AZ], Juvederm Ultra [Allergan, Irvine, CA], and Juvederm Ultra Plus [Allergan, Irvine, CA]) and CaHA (Radiesse [Merz Aesthetics, San Mateo, CA]). The 2 most commonly used fillers for injectable rhinoplasty seem to be Restylane and Radiesse, based on a review of the available literature. Although most investigators do not explain the rationale behind their selection of 1 filler rather than another, several physicians have included explanations for their choice of dermal filler. Becker[5] made reference to the moldability of Radiesse in his report; Rokhsar and Ciocon[6] expressed a preference for Radiesse because of its durability as a subcutaneous filler and its lack of immunogenicity, obviating skin testing.

Assuming safety as a given in temporary fillers available in the United States, when selecting a filler for nonsurgical rhinoplasty, various factors are considered. In our clinical practice, we choose fillers based on their properties of longevity, viscosity, elasticity, and degree of hydrophilicity. We prefer a filler that is not permanent but instead one that is long lasting and semipermanent. Silicone (off-label) and Artefill are the 2 permanent fillers currently available in the United States. Although the concept of permanence is intriguing, it does bring into play the long-term sequelae such as granulomas and additional hindrances to any surgical revisions.

- Two important qualities in a filler are viscosity (n*) and elasticity (G').
- Viscosity refers to the ability of the gel to resist sheering forces.[16] Viscosity is the ability of a material to resist a force applied to it, which means that it is less likely to spread. Lower viscosity products are more easily spread and high n* products tend to stay put, making for more precise sculpting.
- Elasticity is a measure of the ability of the material to resist deformation when pressure is applied. A higher G' filler provides more lift and support and requires smaller volumes to achieve correction.

Fillers with high n* and high G' are particularly desirable for nonsurgical rhinoplasty. Sundaram and colleagues[16] studied the rheological properties (viscosity and elasticity) of 6 cross-linked HA products (Restylane, Restylane Sub-Q [Q-Med, Uppsala, Sweden], Perlane, Juvederm Ultra, Juvederm Ultra Plus, and Juvederm Voluma [Allergan, Pringy, France]), in addition to CaHA and CaHA mixed with lidocaine as per US Food and Drug Administration guidelines. Based on these investigators' data, the products fell into 3 groups:

undiluted Radiesse was in the high n* and G' category. Radiesse mixed with 0.3% lidocaine and 3 HA products (Restylane, Perlane, and Restylane Sub-Q [not available in United States]) were in the medium group. The other HAs studied (Juvederm Ultra, Juvederm Ultra Plus, and Juvederm Voluma [also not available in the United States]) were in the low n* and low G' group.

The n* and G' of each product can be altered by diluting it with lidocaine or saline, an increasingly popular strategy. However, overdilution may lead to the need for increased product being injected at the target site. Being able to produce contour changes with very small volumes is advantageous, so caution is recommended regarding dilution of the inherent product of the dermal filler because larger volumes of injectate may lead to a higher incidence of adverse vascular events.

Hydrophilicity is another factor to consider. There are times when the hydrophilic effect of HA products is desirable. From our clinical perspective, and that of others as well,[17] the hydrophilic effect may be disadvantageous in filler rhinoplasty. The expansion that occurs with the influx of water into the tissues may increase the potential for compression of dermal and subdermal vessels, possibly thereby leading to vascular compromise. Of the HAs, Restylane and Perlane are less hydrophilic than Juvederm Ultra and Ultra Plus.[10]

In our clinical practice, CaHA is the filler of choice for nonsurgical rhinoplasty. Its properties approach those of an ideal filler for this particular application, specifically its longevity (averaging roughly 9–12 months) and its moldability. However, the reversibility of HA products with hyaluronidase makes them attractive to many, especially for aesthetic physicians with less experience in nonsurgical rhinoplasty.

INDICATIONS FOR NONSURGICAL RHINOPLASTY

A well-considered treatment plan is an essential element in any patient's course of care. To that end, a treatment algorithm has been provided in this article to help physicians when discussing surgical and nonsurgical options (Fig. 1). Nonsurgical rhinoplasty is a comprehensive term for the subject of nasal defect corrections. Specific nasal areas of corrective treatment through nonsurgical means include hump removal, deep radix, side wall deformities, tip projection, tip rotation, dorsal augmentation, nasal lengthening, columella retraction, nasolabial angle, saddle nose, contour irregularities, and asymmetry.

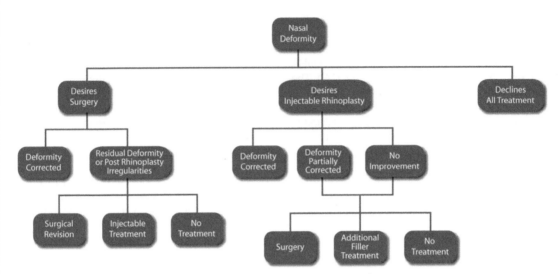

Fig. 1. Treatment algorithm for development of patient care treatment plan.

PRETREATMENT ANESTHESIA

Anesthetizing the nose is an important step in nonsurgical rhinoplasty. If the patient is comfortable during the injection session, they are likely to return for future sessions or refer others for treatment. Topical anesthesia consisting of lidocaine 5% is applied to the nose for approximately 30 minutes. Using 1% lidocaine with 1:100,000 of epinephrine, the infratrochlear and infraorbital nerves are blocked. Rather than blocking the entire infraorbital nerve, the medial branches are anesthetized by infiltrating along the frontal process of the maxilla (approximately along a line where a low lateral osteotomy would be performed). The anterior superior alveolar nerve is blocked intraorally, with the local anesthesia being injected at the anterior nasal spine (application of topical anesthesia to the oral mucosa around the frenulum makes this more comfortable). If no tip or columellar work is planned, the anterior superior alveolar nerve block may be deleted. If the physician is concerned with excessive vasoconstriction of the nasal tip, plain lidocaine should be considered.

INJECTION GUIDELINES

Although the sequence of injection of CaHA (or any dermal filler) varies depending on the deformity to be treated, certain steps are common to all nonsurgical rhinoplasties. For example, a concerted effort should be made to create all entry points distant from the injection site. Distant entry, from a lateral perspective along the dorsum with placement of a series of small boluses (0.1 mL or less), helps avoid tissue edema and distortion of the target site, which could occur as a result of multiple punctures and passes of the needle.

Sometimes, a static bolus method is deployed; at other times, a moving bolus with a retrograde injection is the method of choice. This moving bolus is a hybrid between a static bolus and linear threads, which fills the dorsum from 1 dorsolateral junction to the other, thereby avoiding the dorsum from looking too thin as a result of the placement being just in the midline.

Particularly in the tip or ala, avoidance of injection of a filler under pressure is prudent, in no small part to prevent vascular occlusion. When treating the tip, some degree of subcision is usually performed using the 27-gauge, 3.17-cm (1.25-inch) or 28-gauge, 1.9-cm (0.75-inch) needle used for the injection. Boluses in the tip are very small (0.05 mL or less). The injection plane is deep-supraperichondrial or supraperiosteal. A lateral angle of entry is preferred, but other angles may be used as needed.

Dorsal Hump and Low Radix

One of the most common reasons for which patients present for nonsurgical rhinoplasty is correction of a dorsal hump (**Figs. 2** and **3**). A hump typically comprises bony and cartilaginous elements. Begin treatment of a hump by first injecting above the hump from the superior extent of the hump upward to the radix. This procedure usually entails some filling of the nasofrontal angle. Attention to this area is important to avoid overfilling the angle and thereby inadvertently producing an unnatural straight-line deformity from the forehead down to the hump. A low radix as an isolated problem is treated in similar fashion to a dorsal hump. The more inferior aspect of the radix is filled first and the injection then proceeds cephalad until correction is complete (**Fig. 4**).

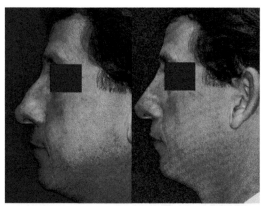

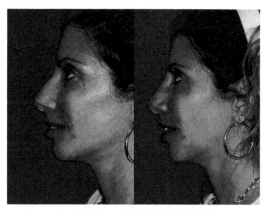

Fig. 2. Correction of dorsal hump with CaHA. Total injectate 0.9 mL. 0.6 mL to treat dorsum and add tip projection. Nasolabial angle received 0.3 mL to treat columellar retraction.

- Entry is from the lateral aspect of the nose just below the junction of the nasal dorsum and lateral aspect of the nasal bone (dorsolateral junction), beginning just above the hump.
- The needle or cannula is positioned in a supraperiosteal plane and advanced to the opposite dorsolateral junction by walking the tip of the needle along the periosteum.
- The position of the needle tip is monitored by palpation with the index finger of the nondominant hand.
- Gentle subcision is carried out and the needle withdrawn to the midline, remaining in a supraperiosteal plane.

Procedure note: advancing the needle beyond the midline helps to create a space

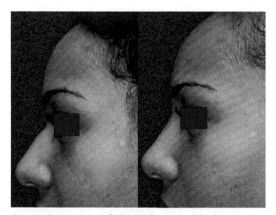

Fig. 3. Correction of dorsal hump with dorsal augmentation with CaHA. Total injectate 0.8 mL. 0.5 mL injected along dorsum and right lateral nasal bone. 0.3 mL placed into nasal tip and base of the columella. Subsequent touch-up of nasofrontal angle with 0.15 mL.

Fig. 4. Treatment of low radix with CaHA.

that allows for the filler to expand to the contralateral side, not just ipsilaterally in the direction of the entry point.

- A bolus of approximately 0.1 mL or less is then injected, depending on the size of the hump.

Procedure note: in general, it is always prudent to err on the conservative side when judging bolus volumes. However, most overcorrections can usually be remedied with molding and massage if the overcorrection is not too severe. Indeed, 1 of the reasons that CaHA is the preference for this procedure is that it can be easily molded into the desired configuration while maintaining its new shape, rather than splaying into the tissues. Keeping injection in the proper supraperiosteal or supraperichondrial plane also helps to facilitate the molding process.

- This process is continued by extending upward from the superior extent of the hump to the nasofrontal angle.
- The correction above the hump is then reassessed and supplemental injections or additional molding are carried out as indicated.
- The area of the dorsum inferior to the hump is then addressed.
- Once the dorsal hump correction is completed, the nasal tip is then assessed to see if there is need for increased tip projection (to preserve or create a supratip dip) or the illusion of tip rotation.
- The columella and nasolabial angle should also be inspected to help ensure that all areas of the nose are brought into proper harmony.

Nonsurgical treatment of the tip/columella/nasolabial angle complex is discussed later.

Dorsal Augmentation

Injectable correction of an underprojected dorsum and platyrrhine nasal deformity is not dissimilar to treatment of a dorsal hump. However, the sequencing is different. Some injectors prefer to initiate dorsal augmentation in the supratip area and work superiorly to the radix. In cases in which the entire dorsum is to be augmented, I prefer to set the height of the nasofrontal angle first and then work inferiorly to the supratip area. Unlike surgical rhinoplasty, in which the preference often is to set the tip height first and then set the dorsal height to match the tip, with injectable rhinoplasty, working from the top down offers a little more latitude to maximize augmentation of the dorsum. Modification of tip projection is then performed and any indicated refinements of the tip/columella/nasolabial angle complex are made. Again, the entry points are lateral, the planes are supraperiosteal and supraperichondrial, and serial boluses are performed (**Fig. 5**).

Some controversy exists about the height of the new dorsum. In his article for nonsurgical Asian rhinoplasty, Kim and Ahn[15] describe the height of the new dorsum as defined by a straight line extending from the desired height of the new radix (level with the supratarsal crease) down to the nasal tip. I believe that augmenting the dorsum all the way to the tip defining point may lead to the creation or exacerbation of an undesirable supratip fullness. Instead, the line should extend from the new radix to the supratip area (**Fig. 6**). In this way, once the dorsal height is set, augmentation of the dome produces not only a better projected tip without supratip fullness but also a desirable supratip dip, as well. If any additional filling of the supratip area is indicated, it may be done after the tip projection is set.[15] In contrast

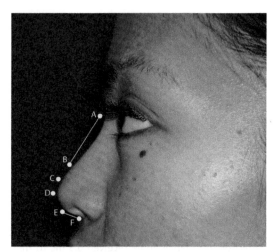

Fig. 6. Line *AB* defines the height of the new dorsum for an Asian nonsurgical rhinoplasty, with *A* representing the height of the new radix and *B* indicating the supratip area, the inferior extent of the dorsal augmentation. *C* represents the new tip defining point, which corresponds with the injection point for increasing tip projection. Point *D* is the site of the infradomal injection to produce tip rotation. line *EF* is the injection axis to produce more columellar show. *F* is the nasolabial angle at which injection produces a more obtuse nasolabial angle, giving further illusion of tip rotation. Injection there should be at the anterior nasal spine initially and then supplemented with subdermal injection if necessary. All injection points can be applied to other ethnic groups, as well.

to Kim's position, I believe that setting the new radix height at the level of the supratarsal crease is too high for some patients undergoing nonsurgical Asian rhinoplasty. Analysis of my Asian patient population would seem to indicate that the ciliary margin of the upper lid or slightly below that may be a more appropriate height for the new radix, at least in some patients.

The Nasal Tip, Columella, and Nasolabial Angle Complex

The nasal tip is an area where good results can be obtained with small volumes of injectable fillers. However, it is also an area where utmost caution needs to be taken, because the risk of vascular compromise of the skin envelope is increased.

- Entry is lateral to the target, with a supraperichondrial (not subdermal or intradermal) plane of injection to minimize the risk of skin necrosis.
- Subcision is performed by passing the needle back and forth to create a pocket into which the filler can be more easily placed.

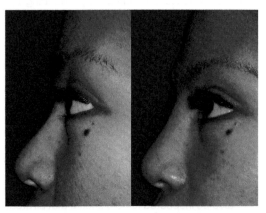

Fig. 5. Dorsal augmentation of an Asian nose with CaHA. 1.2 mL injected along dorsum and nasal tip, with subsequent touch-up along dorsum with 0.25 mL.

- The index finger of the nondominant hand again monitors the placement of the needle. Increased tip projection is accomplished by injecting into the tip defining point, usually in the midline, unless there are asymmetries of the tip that may be corrected in similar fashion.
- By injecting the infradomal area, the illusion of cephalic tip rotation is accomplished. When needed, it can also produce lengthening of the nose. A deficit in columellar show (columellar retraction) is then addressed.
- Entry points for the columella injection are superior or inferior to the target.
- To aid in the illusion of the tip rotation, injection at the nasolabial angle is carried out. For this procedure, volume is placed just anterior to the anterior nasal spine, with supplemental subdermal injection if needed.

Special mention of the treatment of alar retraction and alar collapse is warranted (**Fig. 7**). Alar retraction is not an uncommon complication of surgical rhinoplasty, often caused by overzealous resection of the lateral crura or placing a vestibular incision too close to the alar margin. Although in my experience alar retraction can be improved nonsurgically, this is not an area for the novice injector. Instead, this area is likely best reserved for treatment by a physician who performs surgical rhinoplasty and has a thorough understanding of the underlying disease and relative lack of cartilaginous structure. Never inject the alar rim under pressure. If significant resistance is encountered, either reposition the needle or discontinue the injection altogether. When treating alar collapse, injectors should be mindful that they are not injecting against a rigid structure. Consequently, filling may possibly be evident internally and externally, thus exacerbating any symptoms of nasal obstruction.

Crooked Nose (Side Wall Deformity)

A crooked nose usually entails a concavity on 1 side with or without a convexity on the opposite side. The nose is usually straightened by filling the concavity. Refinements of the opposite side may be necessary to obtain the best aesthetic result. The entry point is best placed distant from the target site. However, the angle from which the deformity is approached varies depending on the configuration of the defect. Again, a bolus or threading technique is used, with placement of the filler being in the supraperichondrial or supraperiosteal plane. Usually, only a small amount of filler is needed, typically in the range of 0.1 to 0.3 mL, but larger volumes may be needed for more severe deformities.

Saddle Nose Deformity

Saddle nose deformities may result from trauma, previous surgery, or septal perforation (**Fig. 8**). If the septum is intact, then correcting a saddle

A

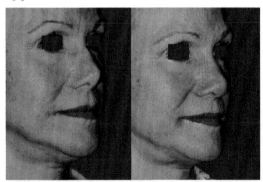

B

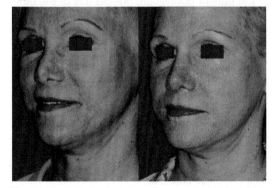

Fig. 7. (*A, B*) Patient status after surgical rhinoplasty times 3. Revision injectable rhinoplasty with CaHA to add length, augment dorsum, and treat asymmetries. Note correction of alar retraction and notching and refinement of dorsum.

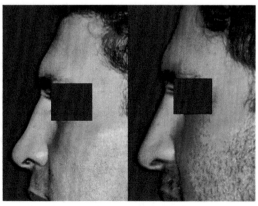

Fig. 8. Postsurgical saddle nose deformity treated with 0.3 mL of CaHA.

nose deformity is straightforward, because some structure against which to fill exists. However, if the septum is perforated, there may not be enough structural integrity to support the filler, thereby making it difficult, if not impossible, to correct the saddle nose with an injectable filler. CaHA is the filler of choice for saddle nose deformities because it imparts more structure and support to the area, whereas HA products tend to spread and splay with little lifting effect.

Thinning and Widening the Nose

Although it may seem counter to reason, the nose can be made to look thinner through a process of illusion. Thinning of the nose nonsurgically can be accomplished by increasing projection along the bony-cartilaginous dorsum as well as the nasal tip. Injecting a filler along the dorsum and at the tip defining point increases projection, thereby making the nose look thinner, particularly if molded properly. When trying to make the nose look thinner, it is important to keep the augmentation near the midline; placing the material more laterally tends to produce the appearance of widening the nose. Conversely, if the object of treatment is to make a skinny nose look wider, then the junction of the bony dorsum and lateral nasal bone is augmented. If needed, injecting over the upper lateral cartilage can assist in obtaining this goal. If injected lateral to midline, fillers can widen the nasal tip as well. CaHA is particularly useful for thinning and widening of the nose because of its moldability.

Pollybeak Deformity

Although a pollybeak deformity is usually surgically induced, it can occur congenitally as well. Postsurgical pollybeak occurs as a result of overly aggressive lowering of the bony dorsum and inadequate lowering of the cartilaginous dorsum. The bony dorsum becomes underprojected, whereas the cartilaginous dorsum is overprojected, usually with some degree of tip ptosis (**Fig. 9**). This procedure produces an unattractive appearance, bringing the superior half of the nose into disharmony with the lower half. When treating a pollybeak deformity nonsurgically, begin at the superior aspect of the supratip overprojection. The dorsum superior to this aspect is then augmented as previously described. Once the bony dorsum is refined, the tip projection is increased to help combat the undesirable supratip fullness. If needed, the infradomal area is then injected to provide the illusion of cephalic rotation of the tip. Any columellar retraction or insufficiencies in the nasolabial angle can then be addressed.

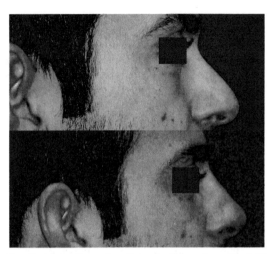

Fig. 9. Correction of pollybeak deformity with 1.05 mL CaHA to augment the dorsum, increase tip projection, and fill the nasolabial angle. Note degree of tip rotation.

COMPLICATIONS WITH NONSURGICAL RHINOPLASTY

Reported complications with nonsurgical rhinoplasty have been few. However, this positive assessment of few complications should include a caveat. The sample size of the subject populations reported has generally been small, with the exception of Webster's experience with 1937 treatments for 347 patients, Kim's report on 87 cases of nonsurgical Asian rhinoplasty, and Rivkin's group of 295 patients who were available for follow-up. Most adverse events associated with injectable rhinoplasty are typical of any filler injection (ie, erythema, ecchymosis, edema, tenderness, and redness). Although Humphrey and colleagues[10] mentioned the potential for nodularity with CaHA, they did not report any instances of this occurring in the patient population, nor did any of the other studies referred to, with the exception of Kim, who described a case of intraoral submucosal nodule near the frenulum.

Inflammation

Inflammatory responses causing erythema usually respond well to steroid therapy, which can be systemic or intralesional. In our practice, we begin with oral steroids (methylprednisolone) to avoid atrophy, which may occur with intralesional steroids. However, if needed, triamcinolone 10 mg/mL or less is usually effective.

Infection

Infection is a potential complication of nonsurgical rhinoplasty but seems to be infrequent, although

Rivkin reported 6 cases of cellulitis. Treatment is with suitable oral antibiotics or topical mupirocin.

Tyndall Effect

One adverse consideration of HA fillers in general is the Tyndall effect (bluish discoloration), sometimes found in use of HA in the midface. Placement in the proper plane can limit the likelihood of the Tyndall effect. If placement is intradermal (too superficial), then the Tyndall effect may occur.

Degree of Correction

Undercorrection and overcorrection can occur. It is safer and wiser to err on the conservative side. Undercorrection is nearly always more easily remedied than overcorrection. Overcorrection with an HA is reversible but not with CaHA. However, most overcorrection can be overcome with massaging immediately after injection.

Vascular Compromise and Necrosis

The most feared complication associated with nonsurgical rhinoplasty is vascular compromise and resulting skin necrosis. There are 3 basic mechanisms by which necrosis may occur:

1. Arterial embolization or occlusion
2. Vascular compromise resulting from external compression of an artery
3. Dermal and epidermal congestion

Arterial embolization or occlusion is rare in the nose but has been reported.[18,19]

External compression of an artery is particularly likely to occur in areas such as the nasal tip and alae, where the skin envelope is not so distensible. Injecting the nasal tip in a patient after rhinoplasty increases the risk of vascular obstruction as a result of scar tissue obliterating what would have been a potential plane of expansion in an uncorrected nose. After surgery, the inherent blood supply of these areas is altered and typically diminished. Therefore, any further reduction in blood flow lowers the threshold for necrosis.

Dermal and epidermal congestion, primarily caused by placing the filler intradermally (particularly in the nasal tip and alae), may not only lead to venous stasis but can produce compression of dermal arteries and arterioles. The hydrophilic effect of HA products may increase the potential for dermal congestion. Usually, compression and congestion can be avoided by injecting in the proper supraperichondreal or supraperiosteal plane.

In my opinion, the most common reason for skin necrosis is compression of vascular supply versus true embolization or occlusion. The 2 main arteries at risk are the lateral nasal artery and dorsal nasal artery. The lateral nasal artery is a branch of the facial artery (at its junction with the angular artery) that supplies the nasal alae and communicates with the dorsal nasal artery to supply the tip. A single branch of the lateral nasal artery supplies most of the ala. Collateralization in the ala is poor, so compromise of the lateral nasal artery or its alar branch may lead to necrosis.[20] This situation is true not just with nonsurgical rhinoplasty but (probably more commonly) with injection in the superior nasolabial fold near the alar crease.

Inoue and colleagues[19] reported a case of nasolabial fold and nasal tip injection resulting in alar necrosis. The nasal tip was injected with Restylane and human tissue–derived reconstituted collagen matrix used to treat the upper lip and nasolabial fold. CT angiography of the patient showed occlusion of the angular artery. Grunebaum and colleagues[17] reported 3 cases of alar necrosis after HA injection, of which 2 were nasolabial fold injections and 1 involved nasal tip injection.

Bellman,[18] in 2006, reported an apparent case of intra-arterial embolization of the dorsal nasal artery after a Restylane injection for the nasolabial folds and botulinum toxin for a glabella furrow. The necrosis occurred in the right nasolabial fold and right nasal alae, extending to the left nasal tip. Although no photographs accompany the report, in retrospect the vascular event was probably more likely to have occurred along distribution of the lateral nasal artery, rather than the dorsal nasal artery.

Skin Necrosis Case

In our clinical practice, the only case of skin necrosis in 9 years of performing nonsurgical rhinoplasty involved a patient who had onset of symptoms 2 days after treatment. This patient had a saddle nose deformity and columellar retraction as a result of a large septal perforation. She initially had injection of 1.3 mL of CaHA to correct the dorsum and tip, with 0.3 mL of that being injected into the nasolabial angle. The patient tolerated this well and returned a month later to have an additional treatment. The nasolabial angle was treated with an additional 0.4 mL placed at the anterior nasal spine; 0.5 mL was divided between the nasal tip and nasofrontal angle. All injections were supraperichondral and supraperiosteal, using a bolus technique. For the initial treatment, a 1.5-mL syringe of CaHA was mixed with 0.15 mL of 1% lidocaine and 1:100,000 epinephrine. For the follow-up treatment, a 0.8-mL syringe of CaHA was mixed with 0.10 mL of 1% lidocaine and 1:100,000 epinephrine.

The patient called the office 2 days after injection complaining of pain and tenderness in her nose. On examination, the left nasal tip was dusky. Some capillary filling was evident but was difficult to check because of her exquisite tenderness. Nitropaste was applied to her nose but the patient complained of burning to the degree that it necessitated removal of the nitropaste after 10 minutes. She was given 2 low-dose aspirin, warm compresses, cephalexin, and a Medrol Dosepak. The patient traveled great distances to reach the office and could not return for 1 week. At that time, there was exudate and some eschar over the left nasal tip and ala. Conservative debridement was performed several times and the patient was advised on wound care. She responded well and had minimal sequelae 2 months after injection.

Treatment of Vascular Complications

There is no consensus for treatment of vascular adverse events. Most would agree that the application of nitropaste as early as possible is beneficial and should be continued for a few days, if possible. Hyaluronidase injection is indicated if HA fillers are used, but there is no standard dose of hyaluronidase. Typical ranges are 15 to 50 units but may be as high as 75 units. Some practitioners recommend warm compresses, whereas others initially use cool compresses. Reasonable arguments exist for either approach. The use of cool, not cold, compresses initially may help slow metabolism at the treatment site, decreasing its need for nutrients. On the other hand, cool may cause vasoconstriction. Conversely, warm compresses allow for vasodilatation but also increased metabolic demands. We recommend treating initially (24–48 hours) with cool, not cold, compresses and then convert to warm compresses, as is our practice after skin flap procedures. Consideration should be given to aspirin therapy (81 mg once or twice a day). Once crusting develops, the area should be cleaned and kept moist with ointment. Oral antibiotics may help to prevent superinfection. Debridement should be conservative to try to preserve as much tissue as possible. Hyperbaric oxygen is a consideration but may be cost prohibitive.[17]

Herpetic eruption

One adverse event with nonsurgical rhinoplasty seen in our practice in 2 patients, but not described in the literature, is posttreatment herpetic eruption. Three to 4 days after the injection, both patients noted the onset of a vesicular eruption, followed by some crusting or exudate as the vesicles open. Erythema usually accompanies the vesicular outbreak. The herpetic eruption may occur in the nose itself or may develop in the glabellar area, even if that was not treated as an injection site. Why eruption appears in the glabella is uncertain. If herpes is diagnosed, then valacyclovir 1 g, 3 times a day, and prednisone, 60 mg a day for 5 days and then tapering, are prescribed. This regimen produces rapid improvement in the patient's condition and may decrease the potential for scarring and dyschromia, because the inflammatory response is held in check. In our practice, we now routinely prescribe herpes prophylaxis for patients undergoing nonsurgical rhinoplasty.

In my role as a consultant, I have seen cases in which herpetic eruption mimicked impending skin necrosis. The patient history is usually helpful in differentiating the 2. If duskiness, blanching, or reduced capillary filling occurs at the time of injection, then the diagnosis of tissue ischemia is easily made. However, the onset of signs and symptoms may be delayed, as it was in the case I reported. Typically, the vesicles associated with the herpetic eruption are filled with clear fluid, whereas pustules may be more indicative of necrosis. Crusting occurs with herpetic eruption, but a significant eschar is more likely to be vascular in origin. Once treatment with antivirals and steroids is initiated for herpes, the response is rapid (usually within 24 hours). In contrast, skin necrosis is slow to resolve and probably does not respond at all to antivirals and steroids. Once crusting has occurred, then the wound care treatment is the same for both conditions. Debridement is not necessary for herpetic eruption, but it is likely necessary for necrosis. In addition, the potential for long-term scarring is significantly less with herpes, but timely intervention is still recommended to reduce this potential.

CONSIDERATIONS IN PATIENT SELECTION AND COUNSELING

Candidacy is based on the patient's desire for a nonsurgical alternative to rhinoplasty, their understanding that the result is not permanent, and whether the deformity to be treated can reasonably be improved by filler rhinoplasty. However, that situation does not mean that the physician should eschew surgical rhinoplasty in favor of an injectable, even although some good fillers are available. Every nonsurgical rhinoplasty patient should be given the option of a surgical rhinoplasty, with an explanation of what surgery may be able to achieve. Likewise, nonsurgical rhinoplasty patients should also be apprised of what injectable therapy does and does not correct.

Patient-Reported Outcomes

Perception is reality, as the saying goes. Kosowski and colleagues[21] published a study regarding patient-reported outcome measures after surgical and nonsurgical facial rejuvenation. The basic premise was to develop a measure of what the patient views as a positive outcome, rather than what the treating physician views. Are the patients happy with their new appearance? Do they view not only the procedure but the overall experience as having a positive effect on their lives?

Patient Expectations

If expectations are realistic, sometimes it is better to give the patient what they want rather than what we think they need. Therefore, if a physician can safely and effectively produce the results that the patient desires with an injection versus a surgical procedure (and that is what the patient wants), then it is incumbent on the physician to offer the patient that option. By the same ethical token, if the patient would truly be better served with surgery versus an injectable rhinoplasty, it is the physician's responsibility to inform the patient that surgery is a better alternative.

Injectable Fillers as Adjuncts

As the patient and physician go through this process of disclosure, one should stay mindful that the changes produced nonsurgically are achieved through a process of augmentation, whereas often the nose may be surgically altered through a process of reduction. Because of the practicality of using injectable fillers to treat minor irregularities after surgery, nonsurgical rhinoplasty can be not only an alternative to surgery but an adjunct as well. Webster[2] stated that injectable silicone, from the rhinoplastic surgeon's point of view, might be considered their eraser. Having an injectable filler back-up available is not a substitute for good surgical technique. The surgeon should proceed as though no such fillers were available and make best efforts to fully correct the nose during surgery. This strategy gives the patient the best opportunity for an aesthetically pleasing nasal result that stands the test of time and does not obligate them to periodic touch-ups.

Not surprisingly, fear is a factor in many people's decision as to whether to undergo a permanent surgical option or temporary injectable alternative. Some have the fear of surgery, others have a fear of anesthesia, and some patients are afraid of both. Many of these patients entertain only less invasive nasal contouring.

Risks with Rhinoplasty and Fillers

With surgery, there certainly is risk involved and no guarantee of the results. Nonsurgical rhinoplasty certainly has risks and no guarantee of results as well. Although particular caution needs to be taken in the nasal tip and alae, the overall complication rate with this procedure has been low, making it a safe alternative or adjunct to surgery. Many people view the injectable rhinoplasty to be more palatable.

Selection of Dermal Filler

The individual physician injector must decide which dermal filler is best for their clinical practice. The reversibility of HA products makes them attractive. However, the rheological properties of CaHA seem to make it the preferred filler. As far as the HA products are concerned, Restylane or possibly Perlane seems to be preferable to Juvederm, in that they not only have a higher viscosity and elasticity but also are less hydrophilic than Juvederm.

SUMMARY

Surgical rhinoplasty remains the most definitive way to improve the appearance of a patient's nose. However, patients increasingly seek out therapies that are less invasive, have little to no downtime, cost less, and have reduced risk, even if the results are not permanent. Over the last decade, various synthetic injectable fillers have become available that now make it feasible to correct nasal deformities nonsurgically. In the proper situation, nonsurgical rhinoplasty can be a safe and effective alternative to surgery. Patient satisfaction with nonsurgical rhinoplasty has been not only high but consistent, with few documented adverse events.

ACKNOWLEDGMENTS

The author expresses his most sincere appreciation for the editorial contributions of David J Howell, PhD (San Francisco, CA) and for the graphic design contributions of Christina Jasin (Tampa, FL), and Dale Murphy (San Francisco, CA).

REFERENCES

1. Knapp TR, Vistnes LM. The augmentation of soft tissue with injectable collagen. Clin Plast Surg 1985;12:221–5.
2. Webster RC, Hamdan US, Gaunt JM, et al. Rhinoplastic revisions with injectable silicone. Arch Otolaryngol Head Neck Surg 1986;112:269–76.

3. Han SK, Shin SH, Kang HJ, et al. Augmentation rhinoplasty using injectable tissue-engineered soft tissue. Ann Plast Surg 2006;56:251–5.

4. Beer KR. Nasal reconstruction using 20mg/mL cross-linked hyaluronic acid. J Drugs Dermatol 2006;5:465–6.

5. Becker H. Nasal augmentation with calcium hydroxylapatite in a carrier-based gel. Plast Reconstr Surg 2008;121:2142–7.

6. Rokhsar C, Ciocon DH. Nonsurgical rhinoplasty: an evaluation of injectable calcium hydroxylapatite filler for nasal contouring. Dermatol Surg 2008;4: 944–6.

7. de Lacerda BA, Zancanaro P. Filler rhinoplasty. Dermatol Surg 2007;3:S207–12.

8. Cassuto D. The use of dermicol-P35 dermal filler for nonsurgical rhinoplasty. Aesthet Surg J 2009;29: 522–4.

9. Siclovan HR, Jomah JA. Injectable calcium hydroxylapatite for correction of nasal bridge deformities. Aesthetic Plast Surg 2009;33:544–8.

10. Humphrey CD, Arkins JP, Dayan SH. Soft tissue fillers in the nose. Aesthet Surg J 2009;29: 477–84.

11. Rivkin A, Soliemanzadeh P. Nonsurgical rhinoplasty with calcium hydroxylapatite (Radiesse®). Cosmet Dermatol 2009;12:619–24.

12. Bray D, Hopkins C, Roberts DN. Injection rhinoplasty: non-surgical nasal augmentation and correction of post-rhinoplasty contour asymmetries with hyaluronic acid: how we do it. Clin Otolaryngol 2010;35:220–37.

13. Dayan SH, Kempiners JJ. Treatment of the lower third of the nose and dynamic nasal tip ptosis with Botox. Plast Reconstr Surg 2005;115:1784–5.

14. Monreal J. Fat grafting to the nose: personal experience with 36 patients. Aesthetic Plast Surg 2011;35: 916–22.

15. Kim P, Ahn JT. Structured nonsurgical Asian rhinoplasty. Aesthetic Plast Surg 2012;36:698–703.

16. Sundaram H, Voigts B, Beer K, et al. Comparison of the rheological properties of viscosity and elasticity in two categories of soft tissue fillers: calcium hydroxylapatite and hyaluronic acid. Dermatol Surg 2010;36:1859–65.

17. Grunebaum LD, Allemann IB, Dayan S, et al. The risk of alar necrosis associated with dermal filler injection. Dermatol Surg 2009;35:1635–40.

18. Bellman B. Complication following suspected intra-arterial injection of Restylane. Aesthet Surg J 2006; 26:304–5.

19. Inoue K, Sato K, Matsumoto D, et al. Arterial embolization and skin necrosis of the nasal ala following injection of dermal fillers. Plast Reconstr Surg 2008;121:127e–8e.

20. Toriumi DM, Mueller RA, Grosch T, et al. Vascular anatomy of the nose in the external rhinoplasty approach. Arch Otolaryngol Head Neck Surg 1996; 122:24–34.

21. Kosowski TR, McCarthy C, Reavey PL, et al. A systematic review of patient-reported outcome measures after facial cosmetic surgery and/or nonsurgical facial rejuvenation. Plast Reconstr Surg 2009;123:1819–27.

Fat Grafting
An Alternative or Adjunct to Facelift Surgery?

Samuel M. Lam, MD

KEYWORDS

• Fat grafting • Fat transfer • Fat injections • Facelift • Noninvasive • Fillers

KEY POINTS

- Volume restoration has become a cornerstone in the current model of understanding and treating facial aging.
- Fat grafting works well to provide volume for the face but may not manage the eyelid area, so conservative blepharoplasty may be needed as an adjunct.
- Fat grafting does not work well for the jowls and has a limited role in the neck region, so a lower rhytidectomy might be required in the older patient.
- Fat grafting does not precisely fill surface problems like nasolabial grooves because it is a soft, pliable filler and also because it is a graft and may not have a perfect take; nevertheless, it should provide an excellent overall result.
- Fillers may be needed to touch up a fat-transfer result to attain the desired outcome.
- Fat is a live graft and is bioactive and can fluctuate with weight, so it should be used with caution in the very young patient, in the individual who has weight instability, and in an asymmetrical fashion to reconstruct lost tissue.
- Using 3 models (a glass of water, a bed, and a house built on sand) can help a surgeon communicate with a patient the role and the limitations of fat transfer so as to adequately establish expectations.

OVERVIEW

Fat grafting, and more broadly the role of volume restoration, has emerged as a predominant method for facial rejuvenation, in many respects eclipsing traditional excision-based surgeries, like browlifting, blepharoplasty, and facelifting.[1] In contrast, fat grafting may be compared with other less invasive procedures like injectable fillers that are office based and require less downtime and fewer anesthesia risks. The surgeon and prospective patient alike may be confused as to the merits of fat grafting and how to incorporate this method of facial enhancement into a larger surgical and nonsurgical practice. This article places fat grafting in its proper place, with all of its attendant risks, benefits, and limitations, within the spectrum of other surgical and nonsurgical treatment modalities.

There is an extensive literature on the technique of fat grafting. This article briefly discusses technique later, but focuses instead more on understanding the role of fat transfer and how to select patients properly for the procedure in terms of safety and efficacy, as well as how to establish proper expectations for the procedure so as to optimize patient satisfaction. This article should provide the reader with a greater appreciation of the pros and cons of fat grafting and how it fits

Disclosure/conflict of interest: None.
Willow Bend Wellness Center, 6101 Chapel Hill Boulevard, Suite 101, Plano, TX 75093, USA
E-mail address: drlam@lamfacialplastics.com

Facial Plast Surg Clin N Am 21 (2013) 253–264
http://dx.doi.org/10.1016/j.fsc.2013.02.005
1064-7406/13/$ – see front matter © 2013 Elsevier Inc. All rights reserved

into the larger world of facial cosmetic enhancement. The emphasis is placed on patient communication using models for improved discourse (eg, the glass of water, the bed, and the house on sand).

FAT GRAFTING WITHIN THE SPECTRUM OF TRADITIONAL SURGERY

As in all other facial cosmetic enhancement procedures, the main treatment goal is to enhance the face in the most natural and aesthetically pleasing way. Another treatment goal is to appeal to the minimally invasive mindset of many patients who shun the perceived invasive nature of traditional rejuvenative surgeries. However, is this a reason to perform fat transfer? Perhaps, and perhaps not. If fat transfer were inferior to traditional lifting procedures, then that would be a weak reason to perform it. However, fat grafting is superior in some ways, and complementary in other ways, to traditional surgeries.

Treatment Goals

After rigorous evaluation of patient photographs over the arc of their youth, middle age, and senescence, I have noticed little gravitational effect on the upper and midfacial regions that would warrant a browlift and midface facelift. In my opinion a browlift offers little advantage to most patients who would benefit from fat transfer. When I lifted their brows with my fingers during an initial consultation, many patients exclaimed that they did not look like that in their youth. When I attended a speech given by my colleague, Mark Glasgold, who showed young and old photographs of the same individual, I realized that deflation was the major issue with the aging process. That realization began my journey to understand aging more precisely, and the more I looked the more I came to appreciate the principal role that volume has in the aging process. Although during my fellowship training I was exposed to a large series of midface facelifts, I have come to realize that the midface facelift has even less effect when volume can be an easy, more reliable, and more aesthetically beneficial way to rejuvenate the midface.

Do I perform surgical procedures anymore? Yes, facelifts for the lower jawline and neck and the occasional blepharoplasty, but both of these procedures are commonly undertaken in conjunction with fat grafting, which remains the centerpiece of my surgical methodology. I have come to understand that fat grafting as a stand-alone procedure can work well to enhance a face in the right patient without the need for other surgeries. Selecting the appropriate patient is mandatory.

Fat Grafting and Blepharoplasty

I almost always perform fat grafting in conjunction with blepharoplasty. I perform a conservative, skin-only upper blepharoplasty in about 15% of my fat grafting cases and only do so when I see that the upper eyelid skin hangs at or below the ciliary margin or when the edge of the skin has a crêpelike appearance (**Fig. 1**). In almost all other cases, fat grafting is sufficient to improve the situation (**Fig. 2**). I use the analogy of a deflated balloon to describe the upper eyelid/brow complex. During aging, the principal phenomenon of the upper eyelid is loss of fat, so it is more analogous to a balloon deflating than a curtain falling. Although it is counterintuitive to a patient who believes that there is an excessive amount of tissue there rather than a paucity, I show them before-and-after photographs that justify my analogy of inflating a deflated brow rather than needing a browlift or isolated upper blepharoplasty to address the problem. I am always cognizant that other surgeons can achieve excellent, natural results with only a browlift and upper blepharoplasty but, in my view, fat grafting makes more sense and it has yielded me more consistent results. As far as the lower eyelid is concerned, I perform this procedure in less than 5% of my fat grafting cases and almost never as a stand-alone procedure (**Fig. 3**). I believe that almost every individual suffers from some degree of lower eyelid hollowness, and a small percentage of those individuals have a steatoblepharon that is so substantial as to justify excision along with additional fat placed along the orbital rim for optimal results. I perform a selective lower eyelid blepharoplasty using a transconjunctival approach to remove any excessive fat from the lower eyelid before I inject fat into the orbital rim hollowness. As mentioned earlier, in most cases fat grafting is sufficient to cover the exposed eyebag that represents an exposed fat pad circumscribed and exacerbated by a hollow orbital rim below.

Fat Grafting and Facelift

The term facelift is a broadly encompassing and confusing term. When I refer to a facelift I am specifically referring to a lower face (jawline) and neck lift using whatever technique appeals to the reader. I personally perform my facelifts through an superficial musculo-aponeurotic system technique and do so only in patients who would benefit from it. A small jowl can be easily camouflaged with fat grafting and/or fillers. However, when the jowl becomes noticeably dependent below the jawline and/or platysmal changes are visible in the neck, then no amount of fat or filler can correct

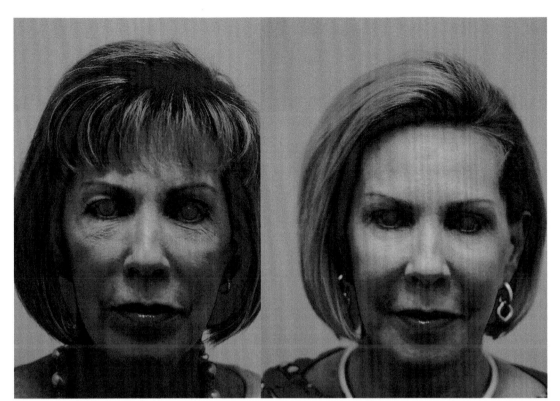

Fig. 1. This patient underwent a conservative right upper eyelid blepharoplasty along with facial fat transfer to achieve the desired results.

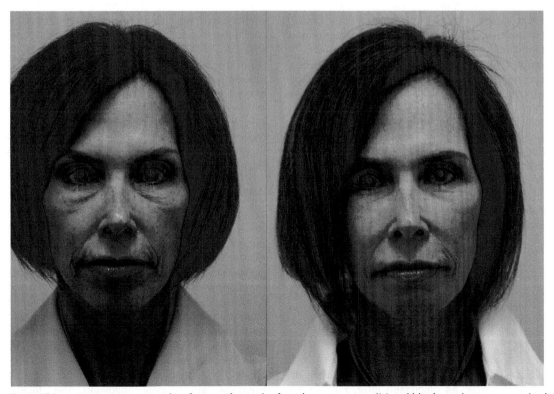

Fig. 2. This patient underwent only a fat transfer to the face, because no traditional blepharoplasty was required to remove redundant tissue.

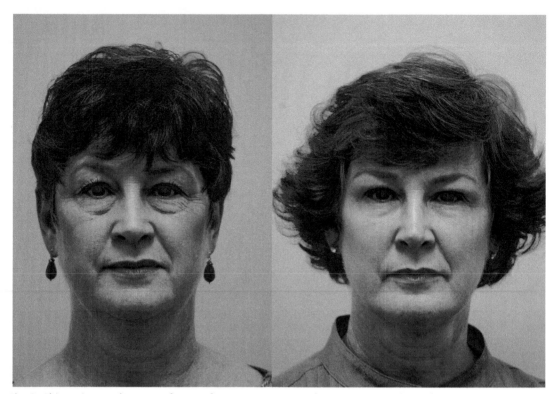

Fig. 3. This patient underwent a fat transfer in conjunction with a conservative skin-only upper blepharoplasty, transconjunctival lower blepharoplasty, and plasma skin resurfacing.

the situation. Further, aesthetically, a lower facelift helps to make a fat-transfer result look better. However, many facelift cases are performed prematurely. Although volume restoration of some kind can be beneficial even to someone starting in their mid to late 30s, a facelift procedure typically is not necessary until at least the 50s in most cases (with the exception of individuals with fair skin, advanced aging, and sun damage who may require intervention in their 40s). Because those who would benefit from facelifts are in a smaller group within the fat grafting group (think of a Venn diagram), most of my facelifts have fat transfer, and a smaller percentage of my patients having fat transfers have facelifts. The exception to this rule is 2-fold:

1. Patients who previously had a fat transfer and have now matured to the point that a facelift would be beneficial.
2. An isolated facelift can be performed in someone who has a very aged neck and in whom the primary focus is on the neck only. In this case, a facelift could be performed without a fat transfer.

Facial fillers can also be used as a substitute for fat transfer, as discussed later. Fat should not be grafted into areas where planned

undermining for a facelift will occur. However, most fat grafting is done in the central face and undermining for a facelift occurs in the outer lower face. In the individual who would benefit from fat grafted in the outer face (eg, in the far lateral buccal expanse or mandible), and would benefit from a facelift and would like both performed simultaneously, I typically would favor performing an optimal facelift in this area rather than worry about not being able to put fat grafting there then in the future plan on adding some fillers to augment this deficient area.

Combined Procedures

To sequence all of these procedures, I perform the lower blepharoplasty first so that I do not encounter and accidentally remove any transplanted fat in the lower orbital rim. Then I perform the fat grafting, which I find to be the most artistically important procedure and one that requires less tissue distortion than would arise after a facelift, which may impair judgment as to how to place the fat. After fat transfer, I then perform an upper blepharoplasty. At the conclusion of the procedure, I perform the facelift, and I may apply the circumferential pressure bandage immediately following the facelift portion of the procedure.

Alloplastic Implants

In general, I am opposed to alloplastic implants as a principal method for facial rejuvenation, especially cheek implants, because of how aging occurs. Both soft tissue and bone are lost as people age. However, in the current era of improved dentition, most aging involves a greater loss of the overlying soft tissue envelope in relation to the underlying bony tissue. Therefore, more bone prominences are exposed, as people age. If this is the case (consider almost anyone more than 40 years of age who has not gained significant weight since their 20s or adolescence), there will be a predominance of bony shadows that develop and dominate the face. Adding hard implants under the skin exacerbates these bony prominences, which can exaggerate the bony exposure and also worsen the surrounding shadows.

The only way the midface can be properly restored with alloplasts is if a greater number of alloplasts are placed to fill in all of these shadows and to simulate soft tissue coverage, namely in the nasojugal region, tear trough, central and lateral malar area, and extended buccal zone. All these implants could be replaced with careful sculpting of fat into these depressed zones.

The chin is another area that I think has been overaugmented with alloplasts. For the younger patient with microgenia, a chin implant is the preferred method to correct the deficiency because like replaces like (ie, a weak bony chin is replaced by a hard implant). As people age, the fat loss around the chin, especially, the area above where an implant could safely reside, namely the mental sulcus region, becomes more pronounced and requires fat or, alternatively, a filler in most cases. Just like a malar implant, a chin implant can exacerbate the depth of surrounding soft tissue loss and in this case it can make the mental sulcus look deeper and the whole region bonier, which is another indication of aging.

Fat Grafting: Patient Selection

Fat grafting is not necessarily safe for all comers. The 2 groups of individuals whom I counsel against fat grafting are the very young (less than age 35 years) and those with weight instability. The reason is the same as for not performing fat transfer in both of these groups. Young people do not know how they will age over time in terms of weight gain. If someone gains significant weight (on the order of more than 10 kg), the fat that is transplanted is liable to grow and to distort the face because it is not a bioinert substance like injectable hyaluronic acid, but behaves like grafted fat.

Because fat is traditionally harvested from the lower abdomen and thighs, it is a tenacious kind of fat (ie, it stays well), but it also is subject to the nature of abdominal and thigh fat (ie, it is the first area to gain size with weight fluctuations). This caution is particularly applicable when a patient has lost significant weight and is ready to undergo a fat transfer. I think that it is almost always safer to graft a patient who either has a long history of weight stability or is undergoing a fat transfer before significant weight loss. I like to undertake a fat transfer in someone losing weight about one-third of the way toward an ideal but realistically targeted body weight.

During my studies for my hair-transplant board certification, I realized that fat grafting in many ways reflected how hair grows after a hair-transplantation procedure. Like grafted hairs, parcels of fat that are transplanted behave like free grafts. After an early period of so-called primary and secondary inosculation that may last a few months, the grafted fat attains a long-term, durable blood supply, or neovascularization. For this reason, transplanted hairs begin to flourish and grow after 6 months but continue to do so up until 18 months. I have witnessed the same changes in grafted fat, in which they start to improve in many cases 6 to 18 months later. The difference with grafted hairs is that, early on, a volume of fat is present that may be confused with a final result. As the fat cells shrink slightly over a period of a few months, the patient begins to fear that the result is dissipating. The patient should be reassured that, in most cases, the fat begins to show slight then ongoing improvement for a year or more after this aesthetic valley, which I refer to as the dip. It does not always return. Just like grafted hairs, there is some variability as to total take of fat. However, if fat is used to rebuild multiple facial areas (eg, temples, brows, upper eyelids, lower eyelid, anterior and lateral cheeks, extended buccal regions, anterior chin, and pre-jowl sulcus), even if the take is not perfect in any one area, the overall result should be favorable. Small touch-ups can be performed with injectable fillers, a point that is discussed more thoroughly later.

FAT GRAFTING WITHIN THE SPECTRUM OF INJECTABLE, NONINVASIVE FILLERS

Many surgeons think that fat grafting has created a major inroad into traditional facelifting procedures, eclipsing many of them for the reasons discussed earlier. Although I think this is the case, fat grafting has also been replaced to a large extent in my own practice by the use of injectable fillers.

With the ongoing trend toward less and less invasive procedures, fat grafting, which was thought originally to be less invasive than a facelift, now is considered too invasive because of the morbidity of anesthesia and the nature of the recovery. In addition to that, the increased use of disposable microcannulas for fillers in the last 2 years in my practice has made it possible for me to perform advanced periorbital filling that I could only have accomplished with fat grafting a few years ago. For these two reasons, I have migrated a large proportion of candidates for fat grafting over to fillers after explaining the pros and cons of each of the two treatments to them. Because these two alternative and complementary fillers need to be clearly articulated as to their pros and cons, I have developed 3 models or paradigms with which to discuss how I view the role of injectable filers and fat grafting.

Glass-of-Water Model

Many prospective patients ask how long fat lasts. When I explain that it is permanent, minus ongoing aging, that may be a confusing point of discussion. Therefore, I explain how aging is similar to a glass of water emptying (**Fig. 4**). When a person is 1, 10, or 20 years old, there is a lot of baby fat on the face so that, no matter how thin people are, they can look too fat in the face. I say that the glass of water in this case is too full. Most women like their face more in their early 30s, when they are slimmer in the face but not yet gaunt or aged in appearance.

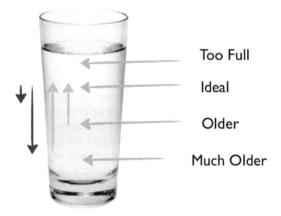

Too Full

Ideal

Older

Much Older

Fig. 4. The glass-of-water model is used to describe how, as people age, they lose volume starting from a point of being too full in our adolescence and early 20s, with subsequent progressive volume loss over time. The yellow arrows indicate the amount of fat to be transplanted based on the relative age, or hollowness. The pink arrows indicate that, over time, there is ongoing emptying of the face, represented by the glass of water.

I call this the ideal water line in the glass of water. As people age (as long as weight is maintained), they continue to lose water in the glass. Someone 40 years old is less empty than someone 60 years old. The person at age 40 years needs less water to fill the glass. When I discuss whether to perform fillers or fat transfer, I therefore say that, because fat is softer than fillers, it takes approximately 3 syringes of grafted fat to equal 1 syringe of injected filler. The emptier your glass is, the more water I need to put in. If I typically put 45 cm^3 of fat into the face, I would need perhaps about 15 syringes of fillers to accomplish a similar end. I then weigh the price of 15 syringes of fillers against the free, unlimited fat that would be needed to accomplish a similar objective. If someone is older and needs even more fillers to get the job done, then the cost of fat grafting by comparison is less (**Fig. 5**). Further, as people age, the glass of water continues to empty despite being filled up to an ideal height. Because the incremental loss is small each year, a little filler can be used to improve matters and to counteract any further signs of aging. In addition, I emphasize that fat grafting is imprecise and that it does not have 100% take or viability. Instead, about 80% of the glass of water is filled with fat and that often some additional fillers are necessary to finish and polish the remaining 20% (**Fig. 6**). The patient can accordingly expect good results with an isolated fat transfer but, after 1 year, when the fat-transfer result has matured, then additional fillers may make the result even better (**Fig. 7**). I think that communication with a patient before a procedure using clear models and metaphors is important so as to limit blame afterward. My favorite expression is that what is told to a patient before paying money is an education and what is told afterward is an excuse. I prefer to offer an education rather than an excuse.

Face-Like-a-Bed Model

I use another analogy to help patients understand the role of fat grafting compared with fillers, neurotoxins, and other skin treatments. I liken the face to a bed that is composed of 3 layers from bottom to top: the mattress, the duvet, and the sheets (**Fig. 8**). I know that traditionally sheets are situated below the duvet but, for sake of this model, they are not. The mattress, which is the deep foundation for the face and occupies most of the bed, is analogous to a fat transfer. Fat is placed deeply, away from the surface, and occupies most of the face after a transfer. However, because fat is a soft material and is placed deeply, it does not alter the surface of the skin very much. When

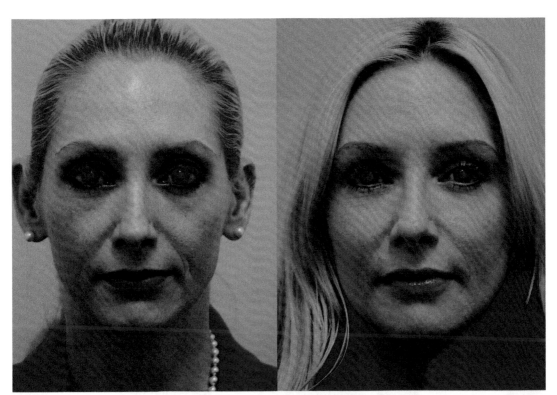

Fig. 5. This individual decided to have fillers performed rather than fat grafting. She is shown at 35 years of age (*left*) and at 41 years of age (*right*) after numerous fillers intended to act like a fat graft.

patients ask whether a fat transfer will fix a fold or a wrinkle, my typical reply is therefore that it will not. It is unreliable to do that. This answer may sound obvious but many patients have said to me that a physician promised them that fat would precisely manage a single fold, tear trough, or line perfectly, or at least that was their perception of

80 / 20

Ideal | ·············· ← Fillers (20%)

← Fat Grafting (80%)

Fig. 6. Using the glass of water to show that fat grafting can fill the face up to 80% to 85% of the result but fillers may often be needed to finish the work and make the face as ideal as possible.

the situation. However, perception is reality, and disappointment sets in.

The duvet above the mattress is what I consider to represent the role of fillers. The medium-sized dents in the skin are reliably and accurately treated with injectable fillers. Because injectable fillers are not grafts, they are more reliable at improving a targeted surface problem. They are also typically firmer in nature and thereby can effect a more precise change in a limited area. In addition, because they can be injected proximal to the skin surface, they can target deficiencies more reliably than fat grafting. For this reason, when someone just wants a tear trough managed, I use fillers because of their lower cost and more targeted improvements. Fillers can replace fat but fat cannot replace fillers; that is, fillers can be used to fill the mattress but cost can be prohibitive if the mattress is empty. In contrast, fat is too imprecise to fill the duvet, or to fix precisely small skin irregularities.

The sheets of the bed represent the skin surface. These sheets cannot be managed with fillers or fat grafting. Instead, neurotoxins are the principal way of managing the sheets in terms of active wrinkles of the upper face because, if the sheets are moving, ironing them does not manage

A

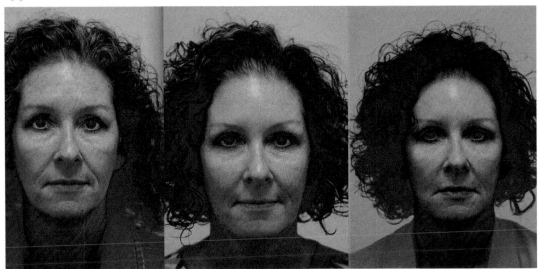

B

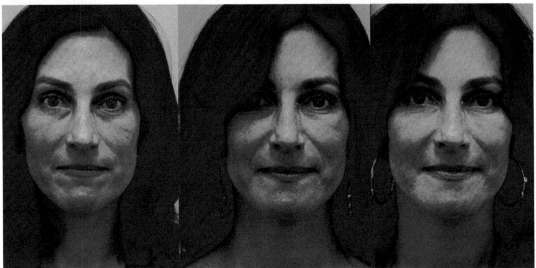

Fig. 7. These (*A*, *B*) patients are shown before (*left*) and after (*middle*) a fat transfer, then after additional fillers (*right*) to touch up the fat transfer result.

the wrinkles in the long term. Only stopping the movement helps to fix the wrinkles over time, allowing the skin to heal. With sun damage, chemical peels, lasers, and skin-care products are ways to manage the uneven sheets, and would be analogous to ironing the sheets.

House-on-Sand Model

I have often been asked whether an individual could try fillers first before having a fat transfer. I explain that this is not an ideal method for several reasons. I say it is like building a house on sand

(**Fig. 9**). When the fat graft sits on top of fillers that are first injected, the fillers are on the way out or disappearing so the permanent fat graft (the house) is sitting on a temporary structure of fillers (the sand). Adding fillers on top of fat transfer is acceptable and, as explained earlier, may even be necessary at certain times to get the best results (**Fig. 10**). The fat graft that is permanent should be built first and then the fillers can be added on top to complete the fat graft result because a temporary product on top of a permanent product in my opinion is acceptable. Sometimes I have heard the argument that using

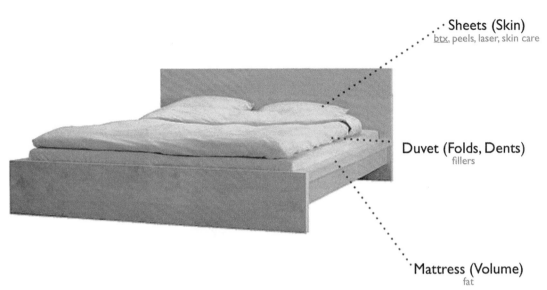

Sheets (Skin)
btx, peels, laser, skin care

Duvet (Folds, Dents)
fillers

Mattress (Volume)
fat

Fig. 8. Using the analogy of a bed to describe how fat is used to fill up the mattress, fillers are used to fill the duvet, and skin treatments (neurotoxin, lasers, peels, and skin-care products) are used to treat the sheets of the bed.

hyaluronic acid (HA) before a fat transfer offers a good trial run because the HA could be dissolved with hyaluronidase. However, this is not a good option in my opinion because hyaluronidase dissolves not only the HA product but also the surrounding natural collagen. Even though collagen is replenished over time, this can lead to unpredictable dents and soft tissue loss that can be disconcerting and long lasting. I typically advise my patients to make their decision early regarding whether to choose fat transfer or fillers and that, if fillers are chosen, then fat transfer will not be

a viable option in the future. There are a few exceptions. If someone has had fillers in areas where fat transfer does not work well, like the nasolabial grooves and lips, then fat transfer will not interfere with the result. In addition, if someone has had fillers in areas like the tear troughs or cheeks that could compete against fat transfer, they could still have a fat transfer later if they have waited more than a year or are willing to accept the risk that they would need to pay for more fat transfer or fillers to adjust for the previous fillers if they should diminish over time. The reason

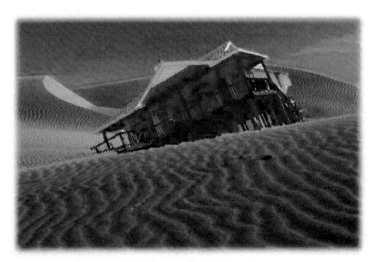
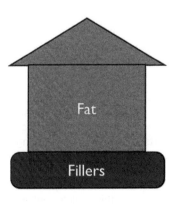

Fig. 9. The model of a house on sand shows that, by putting fat on top of fillers, the permanent filler of fat may appear to dissipate on top of a nonstable, temporary filler, and therefore is unadvisable.

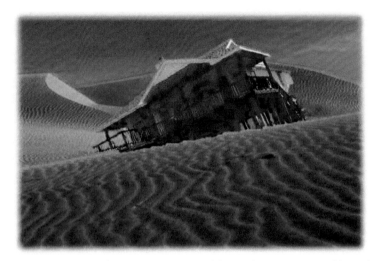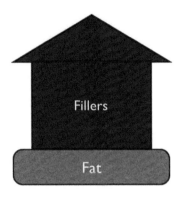

Fig. 10. Temporary fillers placed on top of fat grafting are acceptable and to be encouraged to touch up a fat-transfer result, as needed.

that I typically select the period of a year is that after a year or more, if filler is still present, it will be present for life. I have seen this in my own staff who have received supposedly temporary fillers years ago and have not needed any further touch-ups after a few rounds of injections. In addition, if permanent fillers like polymethylmethacrylate (PMMA, Artefill) is used to inject the face first, then fat could be added on top of the PMMA because it is a permanent filler (fat) on top of a permanent filler (PMMA). However, 2 caveats should be issued. First, PMMA is expensive and, if the face has already been filled with numerous vials, then fat may be unnecessary. In addition, the patient may be disconcerted at the considerable expense both for PMMA fillers and also for fat transfer. For these reasons, it is common for me to perform a fat transfer and add to it with PMMA, because patients like the idea of following a permanent filler with a permanent filler, but it is unlikely that I would use a permanent filler like PMMA and follow it with a fat transfer.

Fat-Grafting Technique

Although this article is principally about conceptual thinking, some discussion of my technique is required. The procedure can be divided into 3 parts: harvesting, processing, and infiltration of fat. To recount every nuanced step is beyond the scope of this article, and I refer readers to my textbook, *Complementary Fat Grafting*. However, this article outlines the fundamental elements of each part of the procedure to explain the essence of how to perform a fat-transfer procedure.

Anesthesia for fat grafting

I prefer to perform all of my procedures using general anesthesia and to avoid the use of any local anesthesia in the donor or recipient areas, for several reasons. First, there is some degree of discomfort that is encountered during both parts of the procedure that can be avoided with general anesthesia. Second, excessive tumescent anesthesia in the donor area can contribute to the outcome of less-viable fat cells, because the fat architecture is altered by robust infiltration of solution. Third, when designing a face, I like to create minimal distortion, which can adversely arise from placement of local anesthesia. Fourth, the infiltration of local anesthesia can contribute to more edema and ecchymosis owing to multiple, additional needle injections.

Fat harvesting

I harvest fat principally from the lower abdomen and inner thighs but frequently venture to the lateral waist, anterior thigh, and lateral thighs as needed. I have also had to use the triceps, lower back, buttocks, and inner knee on rare occasions when a patient is too svelte (or has previously been liposuctioned) for me to find adequate resources.

- I use a standard Byron bullet-tipped cannula fitted to 10-mL Luer-Lok syringes, and I secure the syringe with negative pressure using a Johnny Lock device (Tulip Medical Inc., San Diego, CA) that clips onto the hub of the syringe and that maintains the negative pressure.

- I enter the skin using a 16-gauge Nokor needle through which I pass the harvesting cannula.
- I harvest about twice the volume of intended fat for infiltration, because half of the additional volume is usually a mixture of blood and lysed fat cells.
- If I find the harvest to be particularly hemorrhagic, I may harvest an additional amount to ensure an adequate quantity for infiltration.

Fat processing

Once all of the fat has been sterilely harvested, my assistant aids in the processing of the fat.

- A cap and plug are placed on the respective sides of the 10-mL syringe containing fat after the plunger has been removed.
- A balanced number of syringes are placed into the centrifuge in sterile sleeves and spun at 3000 rpm for a period of 3 minutes.
- The syringes are then removed sterilely and the supernatant is drained from the top by pouring it off.
- The infranatant, consisting primarily of blood, is drained off second from the Luer-Lok side.
- The fat is then transferred into a larger 25-mL syringe to facilitate rapid transfer into 1-mL Luer-Lok syringes designed for infiltration using a female-to-female Luer-Lok adapter.
- These 1-mL syringes are fitted with 1.2-mm Tulip nondisposable cannulas intended for facial infiltration.

Marking the injection areas

I prefer to mark the patient out using Sharpie marking pens because permanent markers are less tenacious (which is a good thing) than gentian violet, which can disfigure a patient for a few days to a week. I use a black Sharpie pen to mark out the areas intended for fat infiltration and I use a red Sharpie pen to make little circles of where I intend to enter with an 18-gauge standard needle.

My standard entries include 3 points of entry for each lower eyelid that rest in the midcheek (medial, lateral, and canthus); at the lateral canthus, to access the brow and temple; and at the medial extent of the jowl, to access the prejowl and the anterior chin region.

I typically like to observe the patient beforehand in the full-upright sitting position in the preanesthesia area to determine the volumes that I intend to place into the face before entering the operating room (OR). I then memorize those numbers so that, when I enter the OR, I have a good sense of what I plan to place where. If I forget, I consult a digital image on a nearby computer screen to remind me of the undistorted appearance of the face. Even without additional anesthetic, the act of placing fat into a face with the patient in a supine position makes it difficult to read in a clear way how much fat should be placed into which areas. Understand what would be an acceptable amount to place in each area comes with experience, and the reader should err on the side of caution, because additional fat can always be placed but it is hard to remove excessive quantities.

Fat infiltration

I always start with the lower eyelid/tear trough area because it is technically the most difficult area to fill.

- The surgeon should use the index finger of the nondominant hand to protect the globe and to provide tactile feedback that the cannula tip is resting in the right position.
- The cannula entry in the midcheek should approach the orbital rim in a perpendicular fashion and the cannula tip should rest just above the periosteum, feeling a release of tissue when the surgeon arrives at the orbital rim. This anatomic release represents the orbital septum being violated as fat is deposited.
- The surgeon should be deliberately slow in placing fat along the orbital rim, to avoid exceeding 3 to 4 mL total per inferior orbital rim. Only about 0.01 to 0.02 mL should be placed per pass of the cannula.
- The superior orbital rim can be approached from the lateral canthal entry point in a plane of least resistance, placing between 1 and 2 mL per orbital rim depending on the degree of aging.
- The same entry can be use to manage the temple, with similar quantities of 1 to 3 mL per side again along a plane of least resistance.
- The anterior cheek should be filled from the same lateral canthal entry point so that the malar ligament is approached in a perpendicular fashion and fat is deposited in multiple levels along the way for a total of between 1 and 3 mL per side (all numbers in this paragraph are per side of the face).
- The lateral cheek that rests over the malar eminence and farther laterally is approached by the initial midcheek entry used for the lower eyelid, and the cannula is passed from medial to lateral for a total of 1 to 4 mL.
- That same entry can be used to place fat into the buccal area, again going medial to lateral with a wide variance of amounts depending

on the severity of buccal hollowing, ranging from 0 to 6 mL per side.

- This same entry again can be used to approach the canine fossa and nasolabial groove depression in a perpendicular fashion with between 2 and 6 mL per side, as needed.
- The final entry situated at the medial extent of the prejowl can be used to fill the prejowl and the anterior chin expanse with between 2 and 4 mL per area per side.

Postoperative patient care

After surgery, the patient does not receive a bandage and is discharged after an appropriate observational period with ice packs nestled in the periocular region. The patient is cautioned that the face can feel firm to the touch, which will resolve over time; that it will be difficult to smile because of the excessive edema and fat in the face; that the chin can look like Jay Leno, the brows like a Neanderthal, the cheeks like a chipmunk, the lips like an old woman (ie, too thin); and that the facial lines could look much worse, all of which resolve over a period of 1 to 3 weeks. I mention each of these sequelae so that the patient does not panic on observing these universal findings. The patient's appearance is typically more acceptable about 10 days postoperatively and can consider resuming social interaction, but this may take upwards of 2 weeks, and, rarely, slightly more.

SUMMARY
Has Fat Augmentation Replaced Facelifts?

Volume restoration has become an undeniable adjunct, if not the primary method, for facial rejuvenation and can work as a stand-alone method or along with other surgical modalities. It is important to understand the safety profile of fat transfer, which is a bioactive substance that acts like a tissue graft rather than merely as a bio-inert filler. The unique soft quality of fat and it being a true graft means that it may not completely correct facial volume issues and may require fillers to complete the result. This article discusses methods for surgeons to understand the role and limitations of fat grafting and how to communicate those aspects more effectively to a prospective patient.

REFERENCE

1. Lam SM, Glasgold MJ, Glasgold RA. Complementary fat grafting. Philadelphia (PA): Lippincott Williams & Wilkins; 2006.

Minimally Invasive Neck Lifts
Have they Replaced Neck Lift Surgery?

Steven H. Dayan, MD[a,b,]*, John P. Arkins, BS[c],
Rahman Chaudhry, MD[d]

KEYWORDS

- Skin laxity • Ultrasonography • Radiofrequency • Neck lift • Cervicomental

KEY POINTS

- Understand treatment goals for nonsurgical neck tightening procedures.
- Determine when a minimally invasive approach is warranted.
- Reviews current minimally invasive approaches to cervicomental correction, ideal candidates and expected results.

INTRODUCTION

The growth and success of minimally invasive aesthetic procedures has spawned a dramatic increase in development of technologies and treatments aimed at addressing the growing cosmetic concerns of an aging population. The exemplary results and minimal morbidity afforded by botulinum toxin type A (BoNTA) and soft-tissue filler treatments has caused the patient population to become increasingly adverse to the downtime and perceived inconvenience associated with surgical procedures. Likewise, the aesthetic provider must adapt to the changing demand of patients and accommodate their needs. Often, the fervor for the latest and greatest minimally invasive alternatives may outpace the promised results, and it is of utmost importance that the aesthetic provider is aware of the appropriate treatment so as to achieve an excellent cosmetic result.

The aging process is often associated with untoward effects on the neckline, including accumulation of fat, redundancy of skin, laxity in the platysma, and ptosis of the underlying anatomy, resulting in the appearance of a heavy neck or "turkey gobbler" appearance caused by an increasingly obtuse cervicomental angle. Neck-lifting techniques incorporating skin excision, lipectomy, platsyma-muscle alteration, lifting procedures, and chin alterations traditionally were used to tighten the neck and overcome skin laxity.[1] However, with the advent of new devices and techniques aimed at reducing morbidity and recovery time, a variety of new options with which to combat the aging neck are available to the aesthetic provider.

Although the future of these minimally invasive options is promising, it remains imperative to use careful patient selection and to understand the limitations and capabilities associated with each procedure when selecting the appropriate treatment plan.

TREATMENT GOALS

In contrast to the varying invasive surgical techniques, nonsurgical approaches are often more focused on the superficial dermis and supporting tissues rather than deeper underlying neck structures.[2] The cervicomental angle is the landmark most associated with improving the appearance of the neck, and is formed by a line tangent

[a] Department of Otolaryngology- Head and Neck Surgery, Chicago Center for Facial Plastic Surgery, University of Illinois at Chicago, Chicago, IL, USA; [b] School of New Learning, DePaul University, Chicago, IL, USA; [c] Department of Aesthetic Research, DeNova Research, Chicago, IL, USA; [d] Department of Gastroenterology, University of Chicago, Chicago, IL, USA
* Corresponding author. 845 North Michigan Avenue, Suite 923 East, Chicago, IL 60611.
E-mail address: sdayan@drdayan.com

Facial Plast Surg Clin N Am 21 (2013) 265–270
http://dx.doi.org/10.1016/j.fsc.2013.02.010

to the submentum from the menton to the subcervicale and a line tangent to the neck intersecting at the subcervicale.[3] Ideally this angle is 126° for males and 121° for females[4] and is particularly influenced by the level of the hyoid bone, which helps to define the jawline. A more obtuse cervicomental angle if often associated with ptosis of adipose tissue in the anterior neck. With nonsurgical treatments, one is primarily addressing the dermal structures of the neck and is aiming at modest improvements in cervicomental angle.

Another goal of minimally invasive treatments of the aging neck should be addressing sun-damaged areas. Chronic actinic changes may appear dry, leathery, and mottled with discolorations. Nonsurgical treatments aimed at reducing the appearance of creping or cobblestone-appearing skin and homogenizing the skin tone can enhance the aesthetic outcome.

In the near future, it is likely that Nd:YAG laser and lipolytic agents may also be able to address excess adipose tissue located in the anterior neck, and help correct the appearance of a heavy neck that would previously have been treated by either direct excision or suction lipectomy.

ALGORITHM FOR DETERMINING INVASIVE VERSUS LESS INVASIVE

Improvement in the appearance of the neck, whether surgical or nonsurgical, should attempt to reestablish a well-defined jawline and a more acute cervicomental angle. However, it is critical to listen to patients and understand their wishes, desires, and their commitment level to undergoing a treatment. For patients with significant submental neck laxity and prominent submental fat, nonsurgical methods may fall short of the patients' expectations, especially if they imagine themselves with a tight neckline and a sharp cervicomental angle. In these situations, it may be best to recommend a surgical modality or none at all. Other patents may be more concerned with the appearance of their jowls or chin position, and this may be best addressed with fillers, surgical implants, and/or face lifting.

Nothing can be more discouraging to a practice than a reputation of not meeting patients' expectations. It is very important to understand the concerns of the patient and to ensure that realistic expectations are established. However, surgery is not an option for many patients who cannot afford the downtime or expense of surgery, or who are adamantly opposed to a surgical procedure. For those with mild laxity, minimal submental fat, and thicker skin, nonsurgical methods seem to offer reliable and predictive integral improvement in the appearance of the neck. In addition, those with crepey, dyschromic, and actinically affected skin will likely need a dermally directed treatment regardless of the underlying neck anatomy. Often this can be offered in an office-based setting, using an ablative or nonablative energy-based device or chemical peel. Successful outcomes are directly dependent on the ability of the aesthetic provider to assess underlying neck anatomy and the desire of the patient to deliver an acceptable result.

PATIENT SELECTION

When discussing a minimally invasive procedure, it is important to understand the psyche and goals of patients, so that the best option or combination of options to meet their cosmetic aspirations is chosen. If a patient uses his or her hands to pull back the neck skin to give a tightened-appearing cervicomental angle, then likely a nonsurgical treatment will not meet the patient's demands. Likewise, if a patient requests a neck lift and expects to have a change in skin texture and tone, he or she will also likely be disappointed. At the core of successful patient selection is listening to the wants of the patient and selecting whether a surgical approach aimed at eliminating skin redundancy, a minimally invasive approach aimed at modest improvements in laxity and enhancement of texture and tone, or a combination of surgical and nonsurgical treatments is appropriate. A successful outcome, whether surgical or nonsurgical, is achieved by translating the outcomes expected with each procedure so as to set realistic patient expectations.

Patient Health Status and History

A review of the general health status, medical and surgical history, medications, allergies, and social habits can reveal contraindications or underlying illnesses that may affect the procedure. Patients with a history of keloids, hypertrophic scarring, and autoimmune and inflammatory diseases should be avoided because of poor healing. Moreover, recent tobacco use is likely to have a negative impact on the expected outcome, and patients with history of tobacco use should be warned of its deleterious effects on both healing and expected outcome.

Patient Medications

Medications that increase the risk of bleeding, such as nonsteroidal anti-inflammatories, aspirin, warfarin, steroids, and some herbal supplements, should be reviewed and possibly discontinued before treatment. Any metal implants should also be noted, as possible interference with ultrasound/radiofrequency devices can occur.

Physical Examination

The physical examination of a patient requesting improvement in cervicomental angle should include both static and dynamic assessment of each anatomic component of the neck. Specifically, attention should be focused on excess skin, excess fat, platysma-muscle abnormalities, malpositioned tissues/unfavorable anatomy, and chin projection.[1] In addition, any asymmetry of the head and neck should be noted and discussed with the patient, because this may become a focus of concern after treatment. The ideal candidate for minimally invasive correction of the cervicomental angle would present with mild to moderate skin laxity with mild to moderate adipose deposits. Moreover, patients expressing concern over superficial dermal abnormalities such as fine lines, skin texture, and pigmentary issues are ideal candidates for a nonsurgical approach.

PRETREATMENT PLANNING

Proper pretreatment planning and assessment begins with standardized photography whereby the Frankfort horizontal plane (an imaginary plane running from the tragus to the infraorbital rim) is kept parallel to the horizon. The full-face front, left and right oblique, and left and right lateral views can then be used to discuss patient expectations, counsel the patient on existing asymmetries, relay a realistic outcome, serve as a reference during treatment, and evaluate posttreatment outcome.[2] Before treatment, the area should be cleansed of any cosmetics or debris.

Appropriate evaluation of superficial neck anatomy is critical to proper treatment selection, and should include assessments of musculature, subcutaneous tissue, bony structures, and skin.

Skin

During pretreatment evaluation, the degree of skin redundancy should be assessed by mobilizing the skin from the underlying tissues and assessing how the skin rebounds to subtle retraction. If the skin responds favorably, lipolysis, radiofrequency, or ultrasonographic treatments should be considered. Conversely, patients with poor elastic response would only worsen upon lysis of underlying adipose tissue.[5]

Fat

A poorly defined cervicomental angle can be exacerbated by excess accumulation of fat deposits in the submental region. This area is especially prone to laxity because of age-related or congenital diastasis of the platysmal sling.[1,6,7] When assessing the patient, he or she should be asked to tighten and relax the neck muscles to help target the position of excess fat deposit.

Platysma Muscle

As an individual ages, the muscle tone of the platysma diminishes and diastasis of the medial borders increases, eventually manifesting as platysmal bands.[5] The platysma muscle serves as an anatomic sling for deeper structures such as subplatysmal fat, musculature, and submaxillary glands.

MINIMALLY INVASIVE APPROACHES TO CERVICOMENTAL CORRECTION
Ultrasound Devices

High-frequency ultrasound energy has been proposed as a safe and effective treatment option for cervicomental correction. Ultrasonic energy is able to propagate through tissues to create selective and focused sites of subdermal thermal coagulation.[8] This wound response induces contraction of the tissue and collagen neogenesis.[9] These devices allow for precise deposition of energy to a targeted depth and plane (1.5–4.5 mm), and can be used to target the platysma lying underneath the skin. The ideal candidate for high-frequency ultrasound treatment is an individual with mild to moderate skin laxity and mild lipoptosis.[10] Results are less impressive and more difficult to predict in patients with moderate to severe laxity and heavy lipoptosis.[10]

Before treatment, the subject is given 1000 mg of ibuprofen 60 minutes before treatment. A treatment map is drawn over the submental region and the patient is reclined. Ultrasound gel is used to provide constant contact, and the provider then does a series of parallel passes over the neck area at varying depths to points of thermal coagulation. The procedure typically lasts 30 minutes, and the patient is able to return to his or her daily routine.

Patients with a history of smoking are unlikely to achieve favorable results because of a diminished healing capacity. Localized areas of edema and erythema are common and usually last 1 to 3 days. Patients typically have tenderness in the treatment area persisting for approximately 2 weeks. Results can be observed as quickly as 2 weeks, but how quickly patients respond is difficult to predict.

Nd:YAG and Intense Pulsed Light

Neodynium-doped yttrium-aluminum garnet (Nd:YAG) and intense pulsed light devices are capable of repairing tissue defects associated with photoaging, and help to produce new collagen.[11–17] Moreover, Nd:YAG has been shown to be efficacious in the treatment of local submental lipodystrophy via cellular lysis and collagen neoformation through submental laser-assisted liposuction.[18] In theory, this application of the Nd:YAG could also have skin-tightening benefits, causing not only a removal of adipose tissue but also a more acute cervicomental angle.

Before treatment, an oral sedative such as diazepam may be used at the discretion of the physician to help calm the patient, as local administration of this procedure can be unsettling. Local tumescence anesthesia consists of 50 mL of 1% lidocaine without vasoconstrictor and 1 mg of epinephrine per liter of bacteriostatic normal saline with 12.5 mEq sodium bicarbonate. The submental area should be anesthetized with 200 to 300 mL of fluid. Two to 4 incisions can then be made to facilitate cannulization of the submental region. Energy deliverance can vary, but is suggested not to exceed 2000 J per 5-cm^2 area.

Following laser lipolysis, the fluid can be removed manually or with mechanical assistance. Following the procedure, gauze and a compression dressing should be applied to the submental area, and the patient instructed to return for follow-up in 7 days.

Complications can include bruising, pain, changes in sensation, scarring, facial paralysis, bleeding, infection, irregularities in skin contours, asymmetry, scarring, and anesthesia-related complications.

Radiofrequency Devices

Most radiofrequency devices work under the same premise: high-frequency radio waves are used to deliver energy through the skin to the dermal tissue beneath, inducing collagen denaturation, contraction, and subsequent synthesis. The result is a tightening effect that helps reduce the appearance of mild to moderate facial wrinkles and rhytids, a smooth skin texture, and a slight lifting effect evident by 4 to 6 weeks, which continues over the next 3 to 12 months.[19–21] Heat is nonspecific and, consequently, radiofrequency devices pose little risk to darker skin types.

Immediate contraction of the skin and subcutaneous tissues is often noted after treatment, likely attributable to heating along the collagenous fibrous septa connective tissue network interlaced between fat globules. The amount of tissue tightening, particularly in the submental region, is subtle, and responders are difficult to predict, but newer protocols are leading to increased rates

of patient satisfaction.[22,23] Radiofrequency treatment is best suited for patients with mild to moderate redundancy and skin laxity.[22]

Radiofrequency treatment is contraindicated in patients with a history of a pacemaker or defibrillator, oral isotretinoin, keloids, or hypertrophic scarring. Patients are placed in a comfortable position and a grounding pad is applied. A thin layer of a conductive gel is placed on the skin. During treatment with the device, constant patient feedback is imperative to a successful procedure. An ideal treatment should consist of a skin temperature of approximately 42°C. If the patient feels the temperature is too hot, the provider should move to a new area or reduce the energy settings. The treatment should be warm, but without a burning sensation. In addition, it is important to maintain constant contact with the skin at all times, as partial contact could cause an electrical arc and subsequent burn.[22] Patient discomfort is tolerable and medication is usually not required.

Downtime is minimal, and patients may immediately return to their regular schedules. Erythema is transient, and patients may experience mild localized edema that rarely extends beyond a day or two. Multiple treatments repeated every month have been shown to be of greater efficacy in patients with deeper or more redundant wrinkles. Lower settings are recommended when treating the neck, owing to the possibility of numbness associated with the great auricular nerve and temporary bumps or ridging over the platysma. Lower energy settings will help to avoid this injury to the great auricular nerve or superficial platysma muscle.[22]

Fractionated Resurfacing

Fractional resurfacing offers a potential way to target and improve skin texture, rhytids, superficial crepiness, and dyschromias.[24] Mid-infrared wavelengths and a chromophore of water energy can be used to target deep into the neck skin. Heat creates microscopic treatment zones at approximately 300 μm depth and 100 μm width.[25] The microscopic injuries cause collagen denaturation followed by rapid epithelialization and a wound response.[24] Patient downtime is minimal, and repeat treatments can be scheduled every 6 to 8 weeks if necessary.

Patients with a history of oral isotretinoin, connective tissue disease, and previous radiation treatments for head and neck cancer should be excluded from treatment. It has been the senior author's experience that Fitzpatrick skin types IV and V can be treated using the Alma pixelated device, without significant sequelae. However, a risk for hyperpigmentation does exist, and patients may be treated with 4% hydroquinone for 4 weeks before treatment. Beginning 1 day before treatment, all patients should be pretreated with an antiviral (valacyclovir), 500 mg twice a day and extending for 6 days after treatment.

Patients are placed in a reclining position and the skin is debrided with an acetone solution. After the neck is thoroughly clean and dry, a smoke evacuator is initiated. Laser settings of 1400 mJ/cm^2 can be used, and one pass with 2 to 3 stacks of pulses at each site is done over the neck.[2] After the treatment, a light layer of topical petroleum jelly is applied and the patient is discharged. Patients should be highly encouraged to apply sunscreen to the treated area.

Patients may feel a discomfort similar to sunburn, but this typically resolves within 60 minutes after treatment.[24] Erythema can be expected for approximately 3 to 4 days, and the skin routinely does not peel. An improvement in superficial skin texture and dyschromias is usually evident within a week, and progressive improvement in the appearance of the neck can be noted over the next 8 to 12 weeks.

Botulinum Toxin Type A

BoNTA, most commonly cosmetically used to treat wrinkles and rhytides of the upper third of the face, has been shown to be a novel approach for temporary reduction of prominent thick platysmal banding in the neck.[26,27] This treatment is best suited for patients with a thin neck and thick platysmal banding. Necks with a turkey-gobbler or heavy appearance may worsen and become more ptotic by decreasing the tone of platysma muscle.[2] Onset of improvement takes 3 to 5 days and typically lasts for approximately 12 weeks before returning to pretreatment appearance.

The same contraindications for BoNTA in the face apply to the neck, and include patients with a history of aminoglycoside antibiotics, curarelike agents, myasthenia gravis, Eaton-Lambert syndrome, amyotrophic lateral sclerosis, or any other disease or condition that might interfere with neuromuscular function. When treating the neck, BoNTA should be diluted with 2 mL or less of bacteriostatic saline per 100 U of BoNTA.[2] Increasing the concentration may help reduce diffusion and better target platysmal banding.

To best visualize the platysmal banding, patients should be treated in the sitting rather than reclined position. Clenching of the teeth accentuates the banding, and multiple injections of BoNTA are injected directly into the muscle spaced approximately 2 cm apart. Approximately 5 to 20 U should be deposited along the band and total treatment should not exceed 100 U.[2] It is important to avoid deep injection into the structures of the neck or below the platysma.

Patients are able to return to their daily routines without any sequelae. Complications are rare, but there is a theoretical risk for neck weakness, and laryngeal or pharyngeal compromise with dysphagia or dyspnea, at doses greater than 200 U. It is important to avoid these laryngeal complications by avoiding the area of thyroid cartilage.

Lipolytic Agents

Lipolytic agents such as sodium deoxycholate and phosphatidylcholine have been shown to be efficacious in the treatment of localized fat deposits.[28,29] Though not yet approved by the Food and Drug Administration, initial findings are positive, and a potential injectable treatment for submental fat may be on the horizon.

SUMMARY

Although the current minimally invasive methods for improving the cervicomental angle have not rendered surgery obsolete, these nonsurgical treatments offer an alternative to patients who either do not yet require or are adverse to surgery. Moreover, these treatments provide an effective touch-up treatment for patients who have previously undergone surgical correction of the cervicomental angle. Further refinement of techniques is warranted to ensure reliability and predictability of results.

REFERENCES

1. Dayan SH, Bagal A, Tardy ME Jr. Targeted solutions in submentoplasty. Facial Plast Surg 2001;17(2): 141–9.
2. Dayan SH, Bassichis BA, Greene RM, et al. Chapter 6: Neck rejuvenation. In: Hirsch R, Sadick N, Cohen JL, editors. Aesthetic rejuvenation: a regional approach. New York (NY): McGraw-Hill; 2008.
3. Tollefson TT, Sykes JM. Computer imaging software for profile photograph analysis. Arch Facial Plast Surg 2007;9(2):113–9.
4. Sommerville JM, Sperry TP, BeGole EA. Morphology of the submental and neck region. Int J Adult Orthodon Orthognath Surg 1988;3(2):97–106.
5. Adamson PA, Litner JA. Surgical management of the aging neck. Facial Plast Surg 2005;21(1):11–20.
6. Friedman O. Changes associated with the aging face. Facial Plast Surg Clin North Am 2005;13(3): 371–80.

7. Rohrich RJ, Rios JL, Smith PD, et al. Neck rejuvenation revisited. Plast Reconstr Surg 2006;118(5): 1251–63.

8. Kennedy JE, Ter Haar GR, Cranston D. High intensity focused ultrasound: surgery of the future? Br J Radiol 2003;76(909):590–9.

9. Laubach HJ, Makin IR, Barthe PG, et al. Intense focused ultrasound: evaluation of a new treatment modality for precise microcoagulation within the skin. Dermatol Surg 2008;34(5):727–34.

10. Brobst RW, Ferguson M, Perkins SW. Ulthera: initial and six month results. Facial Plast Surg Clin North Am 2012;20(2):163–76, vi.

11. Goldberg DJ, Whitworth J. Laser skin resurfacing with the Q-switched Nd:YAG laser. Dermatol Surg 1997;23(10):903–6 [discussion: 906–7].

12. Herne KB, Zachary CB. New facial rejuvenation techniques. Semin Cutan Med Surg 2000;19(4):221–31.

13. Ross EV, Sajben FP, Hsia J, et al. Nonablative skin remodeling: selective dermal heating with a mid-infrared laser and contact cooling combination. Lasers Surg Med 2000;26(2):186–95.

14. Menaker GM, Wrone DA, Williams RM, et al. Treatment of facial rhytids with a nonablative laser: a clinical and histologic study. Dermatol Surg 1999;25(6):440–4.

15. Goldberg DJ. Full-face nonablative dermal remodeling with a 1320 nm Nd:YAG laser. Dermatol Surg 2000;26(10):915–8.

16. Trelles MA, Allones I, Luna R. Facial rejuvenation with a nonablative 1320 nm Nd:YAG laser: a preliminary clinical and histologic evaluation. Dermatol Surg 2001;27(2):111–6.

17. Levy JL, Trelles M, Lagarde JM, et al. Treatment of wrinkles with the nonablative 1,320-nm Nd:YAG laser. Ann Plast Surg 2001;47(5):482–8.

18. Goldman A. Submental Nd:YAG laser-assisted liposuction. Lasers Surg Med 2006;38(3):181–4.

19. Fitzpatrick R, Geronemus R, Goldberg D, et al. Study of non invasive radiofrequency for periorbital skin tightenings. Lasers Surg Med 2003;33:232–42.

20. Narins DJ, Narins RS. Non-surgical radiofrequency facelift. J Drugs Dermatol 2003;2(5):495–500.

21. Alster TS, Tanzi E. Improvement of neck and cheek laxity with a nonablative radiofrequency device: a lifting experience. Dermatol Surg 2004;30(4 Pt 1):503–7 [discussion: 507].

22. Abraham MT, Vic Ross E. Current concepts in nonablative radiofrequency rejuvenation of the lower face and neck. Facial Plast Surg 2005;21(1):65–73.

23. Abraham MT, Chiang SK, Keller GS, et al. Clinical evaluation of non-ablative radiofrequency facial rejuvenation. J Cosmet Laser Ther 2004;6(3):136–44.

24. Manstein D, Herron GS, Sink RK, et al. Fractional photothermolysis: a new concept for cutaneous remodeling using microscopic patterns of thermal injury. Lasers Surg Med 2004;34(5):426–38.

25. Burns AJ. Fractional resurfacing in plastic surgery. a continuing medical education program. 2005(1):6–12.

26. Dayan SH, Maas CS. Botulinum toxins for facial wrinkles: beyond glabellar lines. Facial Plast Surg Clin North Am 2007;15(1):41–9, vi.

27. Brandt FS, Boker A. Botulinum toxin for the treatment of neck lines and neck bands. Dermatol Clin 2004; 22(2):159–66.

28. Salti G, Ghersetich I, Tantussi F, et al. Phosphatidylcholine and sodium deoxycholate in the treatment of localized fat: a double-blind, randomized study. Dermatol Surg 2008;34(1):60–6.

29. Co AC, Abad-Casintahan MF, Espinoza-Thaebtharm A. Submental fat reduction by mesotherapy using phosphatidylcholine alone vs. phosphatidylcholine and organic silicium: a pilot study. J Cosmet Dermatol 2007;6(4):250–7.

Poly-L–Lactic Acid Facial Rejuvenation
An Alternative to Autologous Fat?

Edward D. Buckingham, MD

KEYWORDS

- Facial volume loss • Autologous fat grafting • Poly-L–lactic acid • Facial volume restoration

KEY POINTS

- Facial volume loss, both from bone loss and soft tissue loss, contributes significantly to facial aging.
- Understanding the changes that occur and striving to restore patients to their youthful state rather than removing and lifting tissue in isolation is paramount.
- A multitude of treatment options has been introduced in the past decade to restore lost volume.
- Great advances in understanding youthful contours, both on the surface and in the facial fat pads, have occurred and continue to advance.
- Both poly-L–lactic acid (PLLA) and autologous fat transfer offer improvement in the treatment of facial volume loss. Using each procedure appropriately to bring the greatest degree of satisfaction to patients remains the goal.

 Video of a fat transfer procedure accompanies this article at http://www.facialplastic.theclinics.com/

INTRODUCTION

Facial volume loss has increasingly been recognized as a significant contribution to the facial aging process. Changes in facial volume usually present beginning in a patient's third decade and continue for the ensuing years.[1] The extent and rapidity of facial aging vary between individuals and are strongly dependent on patient bony facial structure, soft tissue adipose content, and skin quality. Studies have analyzed the varying contributions of bone loss versus soft tissue loss in creating this aged appearance with interesting findings.[2–5]

Restoration of lost volume may be performed by using syringe-based filling agents, such as hyaluronic acid, calcium hydroxyapatite, PLLA, and polymethyl methacrylate; a patient's own adipocytes through autologous fat transfer; or surgically placed synthetic implants. Each of these methods may lead to acceptable or even exceptional results in the appropriate hands. This article compares 2 of these techniques: autologous fat transfer and injection of PLLA.

FACIAL VOLUME LOSS: YOUTH VERSUS AGE
Periorbital

The youthful upper periorbital complex consists of a brow that is full over its entire height, propped up by the volume of the brow fat pad. Entire articles have been written and rewritten about the normal aesthetic height of the brow.[6] Often, however,

Disclosures or Conflicts: None.
Buckingham Center for Facial Plastic Surgery, PA, 2745 Bee Caves Road, Suite 101, Austin, TX 78746, USA
E-mail address: info@buckinghamfacialplastics.com

facialplastic.theclinics.com

brow shape and configuration are more important than brow height and perhaps lifting is not the solution to the aging brow in all cases. Comparing photos in the latest fashion magazine shows many examples of models, all of whom are exquisitely attractive, with significantly differing relationships between the brow and superior orbital rim (**Fig. 1**). The upper eyelid also shows a variable fullness between patients; all may be considered youthful and attractive. Some youthful individuals have significant tarsal show with a deep superior orbital sulcus, a high lid crease, and little dermatochalasia. Others have little tarsal show with a more prominent orbital fat component and, therefore, a much fuller-appearing upper eyelid. In the author's opinion, the restoration of the youthful upper eyelid and brow complex must be tailored to a patient's unique characteristics and must strive toward the restoration of youthfulness and not an ideal appearance based on the biases of a surgeon. Additionally, the forehead, temporal fossa, and glabellar area should all be convex and full and free of rhytids in the youthful face.

Infraorbital

The youthful lower eyelid complex consists of a short lower eyelid or, rather, a superiorly placed and full upper cheek. The lower eyelid cheek interface should be at the lower tarsal border and flow into a full convex upper anterior cheek. This natural convex fullness results from the quantity of the lower eyelid suborbicularis oculi fat, superficial fat, and inferior orbital rim projection (**Fig. 2**). The infraorbital area ages prematurely when a negative vector configuration of the midface is present, much as the jaw line and neck age earlier in people with microgenia and a short thyromental distance

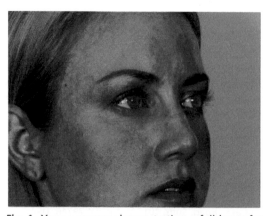

Fig. 1. Young woman demonstrating a full brow fat pad with a soft superior orbital rim and plump support for the brow.

(**Fig. 3**). The youthful lower eyelid must also lack pseudoherniation of orbital fat. The cheek skin should be smooth over the underlying fat and the malar cheek fat pad should be shaped as a teardrop, with the rounded leading edge of the tear inferior-medial and tapering laterally over the anterior aspect of the zygomatic arch. The inferior aspect of this teardrop should create a subtle shadow in its interface with the buccal region that parallels that of the jaw line (**Fig. 4**).

Perioral

Inferior to the cheek fullness, the perioral region should be generally full with a soft transition from the anterior cheek fullness across the melolabial fold and into the cutaneous upper lip; however, presence of a melolabial fold is not necessarily a sign of aging and may be prominent in youth, especially when associated with a full round face. Both the white cutaneous and red mucosal lips are full with associated natural peaks and valleys. The corners of the mouth are neutral or slightly up-turned and there is no marionette line formation.

Jaw and Neck

The jawline should be full and has more vertical height in youth without interruption from jowl formation. The angle of the jaw should have good lateral projection with a well-defined angle that approximates 90° as it ascends to the ramus.

Multifactorial Process of Aging

Aging is the culmination of a multifactorial process that includes the actions of gravity, volume loss, and skin changes due to intrinsic and extrinsic factors.

Periorbital aging

Volume loss in the upper periorbital area leads to exposure of harsh bony contours and the creation of shadows and concavities associated with aging. In the superior rim, this also leads to an apparent descent of the brow. As volume is lost over the bony orbital rim, the support for the soft tissue brow is lost. This effectively raises the position of the bony rim, which is now harsh and skeletonized, and leads visually to a drop in brow height. Illusions of the ratio of the pretarsal skin to lash line and brow also disrupt the normal ratios and offer an appearance of age. Lastly, volume loss in the temporal fossa and forehead contribute, and restoring this area to a youthful convex configuration assists in upper facial rejuvenation.

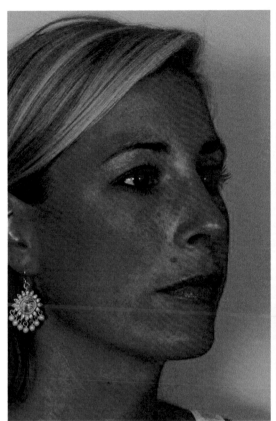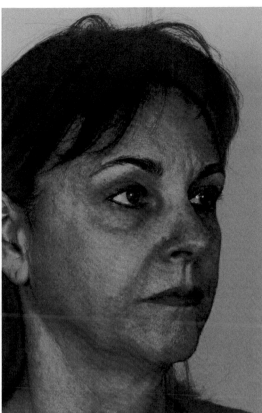

Fig. 2. Photos comparing youthful lower eyelid complex (*left*) with short-appearing lower eyelid and smooth transition between the lower eyelid and cheek and the typical-aged lower eyelid cheek complex (*right*) with a long-appearing lower eyelid and orbital groove.

Lower periorbital/cheek aging

Lower periorbital/cheek aging is perhaps most significantly influenced by volume-related changes and responds well to volume replacement. With

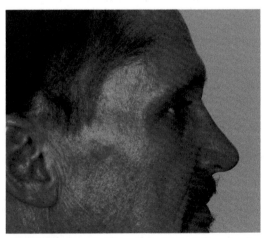

Fig. 3. Lateral view of male patient demonstrating negative vector association between globe and inferior orbital rim.

time, the heart-shaped youthful face gives way to the more rectangular face of age as the loss of fullness in the lower eyelid and cheek region is combined with the increased width of the jawline at the jowl. Additionally, cheek volume loss creates the appearance of shadows as depleted superficial tissues fall and become tethered by various retaining ligaments. Shadows and contour disruptions arise in the lower eyelid and cheek between the orbital fat and the orbital bone. The lower eyelid gains apparent length in this process. Below this, the malar mound and malar septum create a second double contour in the cheek region (**Fig. 5**). Restoration of youth combines removal of orbital fat pseudoherniation, if present, and placement of volume into the orbital groove/tear trough and cheek region to restore the single convexity of the cheek and raise the cheek eyelid junction, thereby shortening the apparent lower lid height.[7]

Perioral aging

Perioral aging results in deepened nasolabial folds and loss of fullness of the white cutaneous and red mucosal lip, with resultant radial lip lines as well as

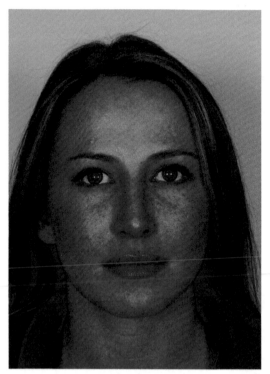

Fig. 4. Youthful woman with full malar volume demonstrating the teardrop configuration of the cheek and the subtle shadow of the inframalar area that parallels the jawline.

marionette line formation. Loss of premaxillary volume, through bony changes primarily, causes the nose to become ptotic and the nasolabial angle to deepen.

Jawline aging
Age-related volume loss also occurs along the lower third of the face with recession of the jawline.[8] Comparison of youthful and aged photos of patients often shows the significant mandibular vertical loss and the appearance of jowling may be as much a result of this change as descent of the jowl fat. Restoration of the jawline is usually accomplished with a combination of surgical lifting and the prejowl, chin, and mandibular angle as indicated.

PATIENT CONSULTATION

A consultation begins by listening. Patients are asked to express their age-related concerns. In the past, patients rarely mentioned that their face had become hollow or that they had a tear trough deformity. More recently, however, patients have become savvier about the contribution of volume loss and often present inquiring directly about its replacement.

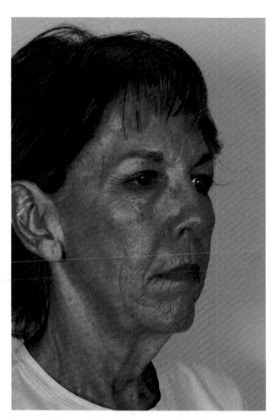

Fig. 5. Oblique photo of a severely aged lower eyelid cheek complex demonstrating the long-appearing lower eyelid with an orbital groove; the hollow, volume-deficient cheek with a malar groove; and double contour of both the lower eyelid and cheek.

Brow Assessment

Assessment begins with analysis of hair-bearing brow height in relation to the orbital rim. More often, the brow is at a reasonable height and the primary factor is loss of the brow fat pad volume and associated volume loss of the temporal fossa, forehead, and glabella. It is only in 10% to 15% of patients that surgical brow lifting seems indicated, in the author's practice. If available, a comparison of patients' youthful photographs assists in the discussion of volume loss and brow position. Often, the indication for brow lift is more related to lateral brow ptosis, creating a flat brow configuration and associated melancholy appearance.

Lower Eyelid and Cheek Assessment

Assessment shifts inferiorly to the lower eyelid and cheek region. First, the presence of lower eyelid steatoblepharon must be determined. An assessment is made on lateral view whether or not any pseudoherniation projects anterior to an ideal convex line to be created at the lower eyelid cheek junction (**Fig. 6**). This is a judgment that improves with practice, but, especially for less experienced surgeons, if the decision is questionable, fat removal is recommended. If orbital fat reduction is indicated, it is performed conservatively, taking care to minimize the inferior extent of the submuscular dissection to allow an undisturbed tissue plane for placement of autologous fat both in the preperiosteal and submuscular/intramuscular planes. Anterior and lateral cheek volume loss is nearly always present to some degree.

If present, festooning should always be discussed. This is a difficult deformity to correct. In its early stages, filling around the malar mound provides improvement, but if a true edematous festoon is present, the fluctuations in swelling may be exacerbated by filling and may take weeks or months to resolve post-treatment, especially with fat transfer. Treatment of this condition is surgical and beyond the scope of this discussion.

Perioral Assessment

Perioral volume loss should be noted, but neither PLLA nor autologous fat is an ideal volume replacement choice for this area. Although the author always places fat in the perioral region with full face fat transfer, and fat may be placed essentially anywhere in the face safely, patients are warned that fat grafting rarely persists long term in the perioral region. It is postulated, much like skin grafting, that the constant movement of the perioral musculature and the lack of a stable bony platform to place the fat lead to shearing of the vascular ingrowth and eventual graft failure. PLLA has limitations in the perioral area as well.

Although it is safe to place PLLA in the cutaneous portions of the perioral unit, placement in the mucosal lip or too near the modiolus is ill advised because of development of palpable nodules.

Jowl Assessment

Assessment of the lower face related to volume involves assessing for the presence of a prejowl deficiency, microgenia, and/or mandibular angle deficiency. As discussed previously, the jowl descent is improved with lifting procedures.

PLLA TECHNIQUE
Preparation/Processing of PLLA

- PLLA is reconstituted with 6 mL of sterile bacteriostatic water and 2 mL of 1% Xylocaine, with 1:100,000 units of epinephrine at least 24 hours before injection—48 to 72 hours is preferable.
- The product is warmed with a heating pad on low setting beginning 1 hour before the planned injection.
- The reconstituted PLLA is then gently agitated and 2 mL drawn into the appropriate number of syringes.

Patient Preparation and Anesthesia

- No marking is performed on patients because the author prefers to see the shadows and hollows without disruption.
- Infraorbital nerve blocks are performed transorally.
- The PLLA is gently agitated by an assistant immediately before injection to ensure uniform suspension of the particles.

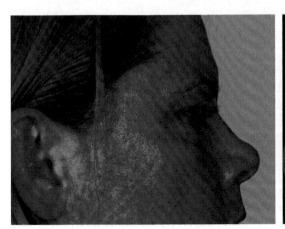 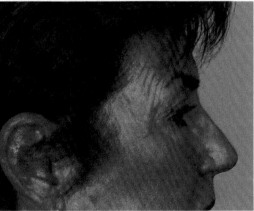

Fig. 6. Comparison of lateral views of patient (*left*) who lacks steatoblepharon and underwent only a fat transfer with patient (*right*) with a sufficient steatoblepharon to warrant a transconjunctival blepharoplasty and fat transfer.

PLLA Injection for Full Face Restoration

- For full face restoration, the initial injection enters over the anesthetized anterior cheek, and the area of the inferior orbital rim is injected, taking care to aspirate before injection. The injection is deep, just over the periosteum. Injections in the central face, over the bony prominences, and temporal fossa injections are deep preperiosteal.
- Lateral face injections over the masseter and parotid or buccal areas are deep subcutaneous.
- PLLA should not be injected in areas of thin skin, such as the lower eyelid or lips, because palplable nodules may be evident in these areas.
- If the product cannot be adequately delivered superiorly into the orbital hollow, more superior filling is performed at a later date with a hyaluronic acid product.
- Injection then progresses from the anterior cheek to the lateral cheek, building the convexity to full correction and eliminating the concave malar groove. Because the injection contains Xylocaine, subsequent needle punctures should be performed, when possible, from treated areas.
- The premaxillary area is then filled as a deep injection and the buccal area in a subcutaneous fashion blending with the malar cheek.
- Injection then progresses to the temporal fossa. Again, this injection is deep and preperiosteal, when possible, but deep to the deep temporal fascia otherwise. Injection in this area is in boluses, taking care to aspirate preinjection. Again, full correction is the desired endpoint.
- The lateral brow is also filled at this time.
- If desired, the medial brow and glabellar area can be filled, but due to the deep locations of the supraorbital and supratrochlear neurovascular bundles, the injection in this area is subcutaneous.
- The lower third of the face is addressed with preperiosteal injection in the prejowl sulcus

A

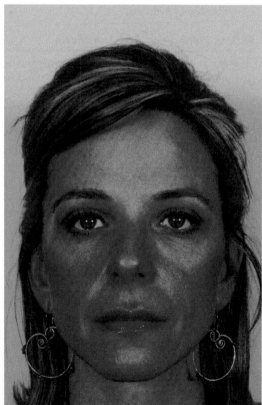 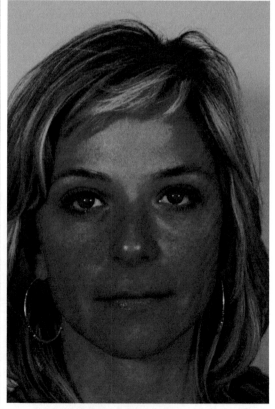

Fig. 7. 44-year-old woman, frontal (*A*) and oblique (*B*) photos before and after 3 treatments, 2 vials each, PLLA to temples, cheeks, marionette, and prejowl sulcus. Patient had overprojecting maxilla to malar area. Note in frontal view the soft appearance of face and smooth transitions with improvement in the submalar area. Note especially in oblique view the distal cheek contour improvements.

B

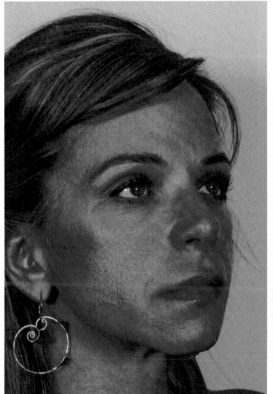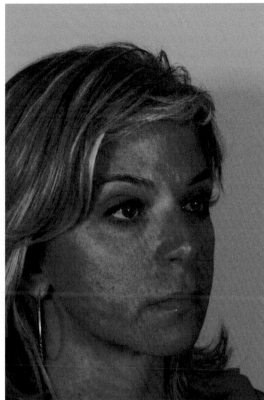

Fig. 7. (*continued*)

and as a bolus, avoiding the facial artery and mental foramen.
- The lateral mandibular area may then be filled in a deep subcutaneous plane over the parotid fascia.
- The marionette area is a subcutaneous injection and, if indicated, the anterior mandible is again a deep injection.

Massage After Injections

- After injection, the face should be aggressively massaged to disperse the particles evenly.
- Massage is usually performed as each area is injected and again over the entire face once the procedure is complete.

Potential Sequelae of Injections

- Because the injection contains Xylocaine with epinephrine, mottled blanching is normal, as is transient motor nerve dysfunction.
- If eye closure is affected, reassure the patient and instruct in manual eye closure until this effect of local anesthetic resolves.

Timing for Multiple PLLA Injection Sessions

- PLLA is injected in 2 to 3 or more sessions, spaced at least 4 weeks apart. As the final endpoint is approached, longer intervals are recommended.
- Although full correction at each session is the endpoint, this is only temporary hydration. Patients need to be counseled that the effect regresses in 1 to 2 days. The PLLA particles then stimulate collagen production, creating lasting volume.
- Incremental correction is achieved with each injection, and variation of response occurs between patients. In some patients, a planned third session is canceled as result of an adequate result from the second session. Other patients might require a smaller fourth session to complete the correction.
- As the endpoint is approached, it is appropriate to delay further injections up to 3 months to avoid overcorrection and allow completion of the stimulatory process.

The published longevity of PLLA is 23 months, but the results likely persist beyond this time. (**Fig. 7**).

AUTOLOGOUS FAT TECHNIQUE
Anesthesia

- Autologous fat transfer is usually performed in an operating room under intravenous sedation supplemented with local anesthesia. Small secondary procedures may be performed under local anesthesia only.
- Skin resurfacing and lower eyelid blepharoplasty are performed before fat transfer, if indicated.

Donor Area Preparation

- Donor areas are marked out in the preoperative holding area with the patient standing. The abdominal area is the first choice of donor area, if available, followed by the medial and lateral thigh.[9–12]
- In the operating room and under sedation, the donor areas are infiltrated with 1% Xylocaine with 1:100,000 units of epinephrine mixed 1:1 with injectable 0.9% saline.
- The injection is performed with a 20-mL syringe and a 3-in × 25-gauge spinal needle. For the abdominal area, approximately 30 mL to 40 mL of solution is injected. Injection is placed in the immediate subcutaneous space and the prefascia space.

Note: No injection is placed in the midcutaneous plane where the fat is to be harvested, to minimize possible toxicity to adipocytes from the Xylocaine.

- Usually a minimum of 100 mL is harvested for full face transfer and up to 140 mL if the fat is of poor quality.

Fat Harvesting and Preparation

- Harvesting is performed with a small 15-blade entry point placed appropriately for the donor site.
- A bullet-tip 3-mm × 15-cm "Tenard type" cannula (Tulip Medical Products) is used for harvesting with a 10-mL syringe.
- Gentle (2–3 cm) aspiration pressure is used to prevent lipolysis.
- The harvested fat is then transferred into the PureGraft System (Cytori Therapeutics) (Fig. 8).
- The fat is rinsed and drained twice within the system with equal quantities of lactated Ringer solution.
- The fat is allowed to drain for a minimum of 3 minutes.
- Concentrated fat is then transferred to 1-mL injection syringes.
- Three different injection cannulas are used:

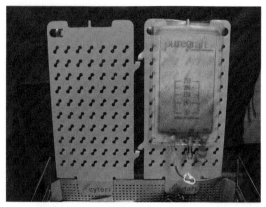

Fig. 8. Photo of the PureGraft fat purification system from Cytori Therapeutics.

1. 1.2-mm × 6-cm Spoon-tip cannulas (Tulip Medical Products)
2. 0.9-mm × 4-cm Spoon-tip cannulas (Tulip Medical Products)
3. Donofrio 16-gauge (Byron Medical) straight blunt cannula (Fig. 9)

Fat Transfer

See the video of fat transfer procedure accompanying this article at: http://www.facialplastic.the clinics.com/.

- Transfer is begun by infiltrating the entry sites with a small wheel of 1% Xylocaine with 1:100,000 units of epinephrine and by performing nerve blocks of the supraorbital, infraorbital, and mental nerve foramen.
- In general, fat is placed from entry points perpendicular to the desired area of placement.
- Transfer is begun in the inferior orbital rim area.
- An 18-gauge needle is used to make an entry site at the level of the nasal ala lateral to the nasolabial crease.
- The orbital rim is approached from below; the nondominant hand is used to place a finger just inside the orbital rim and the 1.2-mm

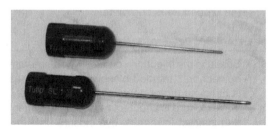

Fig. 9. 1.2-mm and 0.9-mm Tulip cannulas.

cannula tip is bounced off the finger while dispensing small quantities of fat with multiple small passes in a plane immediately above the periosteum (**Fig. 10**).

- The medial orbital rim is treated first, followed by the lateral rim. 1 mL of fat is placed in each location, medial and lateral. A third 1 mL of fat is then dispensed along the entire inferior orbital rim. Less quantity is rarely used in this location and more may be added if needed. Often, the 0.9-mm cannula is used to add fat into a slightly more superficial location to further augment the area.

Note: Quantities as large as 6 mL per side have been placed in this area, but more experience and care are indicated with these larger quantities because the risk of contour irregularities increases substantially.

The lateral canthal area is next treated with an entry site in the crow's feet rhytids (**Fig. 11**). The 1.2-mm cannula is again used to infiltrate 1 mL to 2 mL of fat, blending it in with the inferior orbital rim fat.

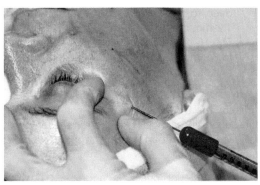

Fig. 11. The lateral canthus is approached from the crow's feet area; 1 mL to 2 mL is blended into the lateral inferior orbital rim injection and toward the superior orbital rim.

The superior orbital rim is then addressed by 1 or 2 entry sites in the forehead, again placing the nondominant hand index finger just inside the rim and bouncing the cannula off the finger while slowly placing fat.

Note: Fat is placed in the plane just above the periosteum if no brow lift has been performed. It is placed in the deep subcutaneous space if the subperiosteal plane has been violated (**Fig. 12**).

- Usually, 2 mL is placed along the superior orbital rim.
- Fat is also infiltrated in a superficial subcutaneous plane in the forehead and glabella and, if indicated, into the upper eyelid sulcus.

Note: The preceding is an advanced technique and should be introduced only after sufficient experience has been gained.

- The temporal area is then blended in with the other periorbital areas with 1 mL to 3 mL of fat

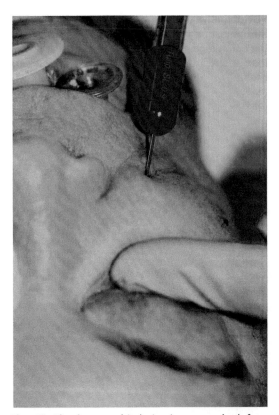

Fig. 10. The lower orbital rim is approached from inferiorly using the 1.2-mm and 0.8-mm Tulip cannulas. The fat is injected in small parcels just above the periosteum with the nondominant index finger as a guide just inside the orbital rim.

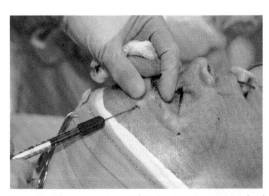

Fig. 12. The superior orbital rim is approached perpendicularly from the forehead. It is injected much like the inferior orbital rim with the nondominant hand just inside the rim, but smaller volumes are usually used.

deep to the deep temporal fascia with the 1.2-mm cannula.

- The 16-gauge Donofrio cannula is then used to complete the transfer except in the mucosal lip where the 0.9-mm cannula is again used.

Note: The Donofrio cannula is less fragile than the spoon-tip cannulas, so the remainder of the injections can be performed with more ease and at a faster pace.

- The anterior cheek is addressed next by placing the nondominant index finger along the lateral aspect of the nasolabial fold mound.
- The cannula is then inserted via the crow's feet entry site and 2 mL to 3 mL of fat is placed throughout the anterior cheek in superficial, mid, and deep cutaneous planes overlying the hollow of the malar groove.
- The lateral cheek is then addressed by utilizing the medial cheek entry site.

Note: The lateral extent of the anterior cheek augmentation is easily visualized. The lateral cheek is slowly built out from this point, injecting in multiple planes and tapering the malar eminence to a point over the zygomatic arch. This should create a teardrop appearance with the tapering superior aspect of the tear superior-lateral and a shadow under the lateral cheek, which parallels the jawline (**Fig. 13**).

Note: Usually 2 mL to 3 mL is injected in the lateral cheek area. Larger volumes may be used for all these sites; the volumes given are conservative and generate substantial results with minimal risk.

- 1–2 mL is then placed deep over the precanine fossa and base of the pyriform aperature.
- 1–2 mL is placed subcutaneous in the nasolabial fold.
- 1 mL is placed in the cutaneous lip.
- 2 mL is placed preperiosteal in the prejowl sulcus.
- 2 mL is placed subcutaneous for the marionette line.
- 0.5 mL to 1 mL is then placed in each mucosal lip, taking care not to obliterate the midline depression of the lower lip.

Note: All volumes quoted are unilateral.

POSTOPERATIVE PATIENT CARE

Postoperatively, patients are asked to sleep with the head upright and apply ice generously over the entire face. No wound care is necessary other than a small dab of ointment over the insertion sites.

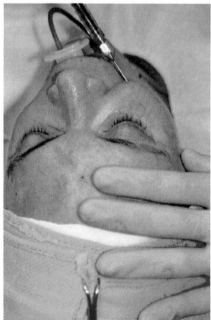

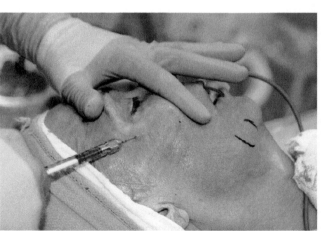

Fig. 13. The anterior cheek is approached from the crow's feet entry site. (*left*) The nondominant index finger is laid against the bulge of the nasolabial fold and fat is injected in the deep subcutaneous and intramuscular plane all along this area. The lateral cheek is then approached from anteriorly (*right*) building on the lateral edge of the anterior cheek fat deposit to form a tapered teardrop.

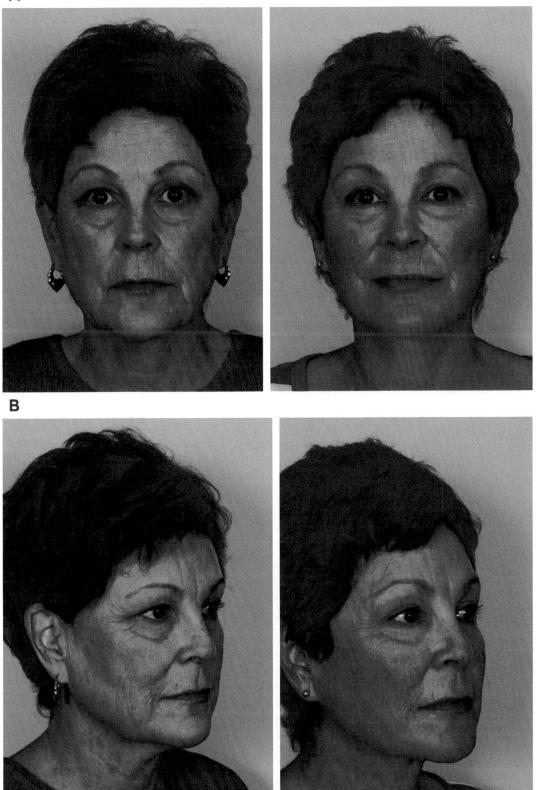

Fig. 14. 65-year-old woman, frontal (*A*) and oblique views (*B*), 2 years after full face fat transfer, full face chemical peel, Upper blepharolplasty and lower facelift.

282

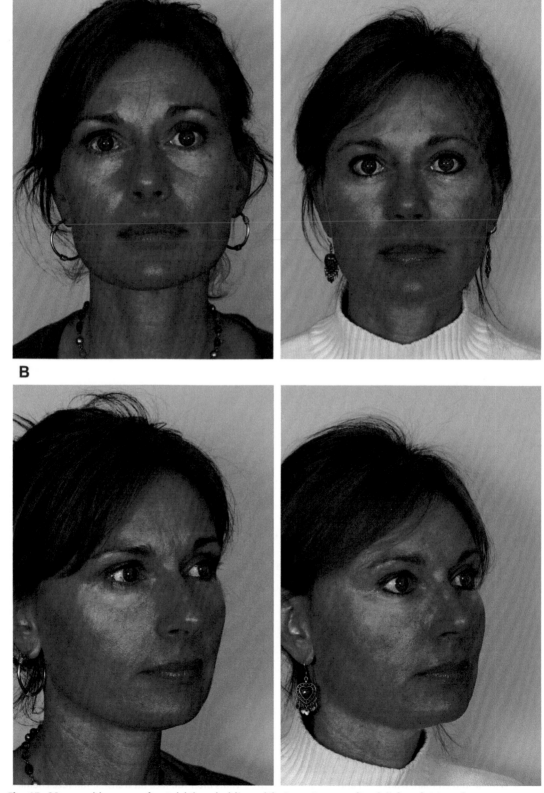

Fig. 15. 38-year-old woman, frontal (*A*) and oblique (*B*) views, 2-years after full face fat transfer.

Patients experience a variable amount of bruising but a consistent amount of swelling. Patients are told to expect significant disfiguring swelling the first week, which decreases substantially by the end of the second week. Return to social activities can be achieved by the end of the second week in most patients and the third week in all.

Some volume reduction occurs through the sixth week and a small amount of volume may be lost between 6 and 12 weeks. The volume stabilizes beyond this time period and long-term results can be expected except in the perioral region (**Figs. 14 and 15**).[13–15]

CHOOSING PLLA VERSUS FAT

In the author's practice, PLLA and fat are the primary choices for full face volume restoration. Although both procedures may be used for regional placement, the author finds that patients with isolated regional deficiencies often desire immediate corrections and choose products other than PLLA or fat.

Autologous fat has the benefit of requiring only 1 procedure, but it requires an anesthetic and 2 to 3 weeks of social recovery. PLLA requires several treatment sessions but is usually performed under local anesthesia only.

Usually PLLA has little to no postoperative bruising or swelling and while it can be used in conjunction with a surgical procedure; most patients choose autologous fat when having concurrent surgical procedures because they are recovering from other procedures, they do not need several treatment sessions, and autologous fat affords greater longevity. Usually if patients are interested in isolated volume augmentation without other surgical procedures, PLLA is used; however, certain patients desire the potential for greater longevity and the soft nature of fat and choose to have fat grafting as an isolated procedure.

PLLA is not advised in the thin lower eyelid skin, but a hyaluronic acid product can be combined with PLLA to accomplish that goal. Autologous fat provides natural results for the thin lower eyelid skin and can also be used in the upper orbital sulcus, whereas PLLA is not advised. The surgeon's role is to explain the indications, risks, benefits, and alternatives of the available procedures and let patients choose, with appropriate guidance. **Table 1** summarizes the comparison of procedures.

GENERAL CONSIDERATIONS

Autologous fat transfer has been criticized by some surgeons for having a lack of longevity, lack of predictability, and potential for irregularities, especially in the lower eyelid region. Although the author agrees that fat transfer is predictably unreliable for treatment of the perioral area, he has had success and reliability elsewhere in the face and has had patients with consistent volume retention more than 5 years after the procedure. Patients do need to be counseled preoperatively regarding the varying survival of autologous fat but the author finds that even patients with less than average survival of transferred fat are satisfied with their results and that few secondary procedures are performed.

Autologous fat offers replacement of like tissue and is soft and natural in its appearance. PLLA, when used to gain the same degree of correction, can at times feel somewhat firm and stiff.

Autologous fat techniques vary between surgeons without clear superiority in many cases.[16] The author implemented use of the PureGraft

Table 1
PLLA versus autologous fat

	PLLA	Autologous Fat	Notes
# of Treatments	2–4	1	Touch-up possible with fat but uncommon
Anesthesia required	Local only	Usually intravenous sedation	
Concurrent surgery	*	****	If anesthesia and recovery, then prefer fat
Donor fat available	*	****	PLLA, if no donor fat
Perioral usefulness	***	*	Fat not reliable, PLLA no mucosal use
Isolated regional placement	**	**	Both, but more preparation for fat
Lower eyelid placement	No	****	Fat desirable
Result predictability	***	***	Both variable to extent
Result longevity	**	****	Fat better longevity
Complication risk	****	****	Both rare

* indicates least beneficial and **** indicates most beneficial.

System approximately 28 months and believes that it has added consistency to outcomes. With the previous use of centrifugation, some poorer quality harvested fat was difficult to predict. A recent presentation by Glasgold (American Academy of Facial Plastic and Reconstructive Surgery 2012 fall meeting) seems to support this, but more evidence needs to be gathered.

Many exciting advances in autologous fat transfer and stem cell therapy are under investigation and promise increasingly reliable results in the future.[17]

SUMMARY

Facial volume loss both from bone loss and soft tissue loss contributes significantly to facial aging. Understanding the changes that occur and striving to restore patients to their youthful state, rather than removing and lifting tissue in isolation, are paramount. Fortunately, many treatment options have been introduced in the past decade to restore lost volume, and great advances in understanding of youthful contours, both on the surface and in the facial fat pads, has occurred and continues to advance. Both PLLA and autologous fat transfer offer improvement in the treatment of facial volume loss. Using each procedure appropriately to bring the greatest degree of satisfaction to patients remains the goal.

SUPPLEMENTARY DATA

Supplementary data related to this article can be found online at http://dx.doi.org/10.1016/j.fsc.2013.02.007.

REFERENCES

1. Ciuci PM, Obagi S. Rejuvenation of the periorbital complex with autologous fat transfer: current therapy. J Oral Maxillofac Surg 2008;66(8):1686–93.
2. Shaw RB, Katzel EB, Koltz PF, et al. Aging of the mandible and its aesthetic implicatioins. Plast Reconstr Surg 2010;125(1):332–42.
3. Shaw RB, Kahn DM. Aging of the Midface bony elements: a three-dimensional computed tomographic study. Plast Reconstr Surg 2007;119(2):675–81.
4. Donofrio LM. Fat distribution: a morphologic study of the aging face. Dermatol Surg 2000;26(12):1107–12.
5. Rohrick RJ, Pessa JE, Ristow B. The youthful cheek and the deep medial fat compartment. Plast Reconstr Surg 2008;121(6):2107–12.
6. Gunter JP, Antrobus SD. Aesthetic analysis of the eyebrows. Plast Reconstr Surg 1997;99(7):1808–16.
7. Lambros V. Observations on periorbital and midface aging. Plast Reconstr Surg 2007;120(5):1367–76.
8. Lambros V. Models of facial aging and implications for treatment. Clin Plast Surg 2008;35(3):319–27.
9. Donofrio LM. Techniques in fat grafting. Aesthet Surg J 2008;28(6):681–7.
10. Coleman SR. Facial augmentation with structural fat grafting. Clin Plast Surg 2006;33(4):567–77.
11. Obagi S. Specific techniques for fat transfer. Facial Plast Surg Clin North Am 2008;16(4):401–7, v.
12. Lam SM, Glasgold MJ, Glasgold RA. Complementary fat grafting. Philadelphia (PA): Wolters Kluwer, Lippincott Willaims and Wilkins; 2007.
13. Coleman SR. Structural fat grafting: more than a permanent filler. Plast Reconstr Surg 2006;118(Suppl 3):108S–20S.
14. Coleman SR. Structural fat grafting. St Louis (MO): Quality Medical Publishing, Inc; 2004.
15. Glasgold RA, Glasgold MJ, Lam SM. Complications following fat transfer. Oral Maxillofac Surg Clin North Am 2009;21(1):53–8, vi.
16. Phanette G, Brown SA, Oni G, et al. Fat grafting: evidence-based review on autologous fat harvesting, processing, reinjection, and storage. Plast Reconstr Surg 2012;130(1):249–58.
17. Butala P, Hazen A, Szpalski C, et al. Endogenous stem cell therapy enhances fat graft survival. Plast Reconstr Surg 2012;130(2):293–306.

Cosmetic Botulinum Toxin
Has It Replaced More Invasive Facial Procedures?

Myriam Loyo, MD[a], Theda C. Kontis, MD[a,b],*

KEYWORDS

- Botulinum toxin • Chemical browlift • Oral commissure • Platysmal banding • Necklift • Liplift
- Hypertrophic orbicularis oculi

KEY POINTS

- By understanding the opposing pull of the muscles of facial expression, neurotoxin injections can be precisely placed to enhance certain facial features.
- Neurotoxin injections, either alone or in combination with filler agents, have probably replaced open procedures for elevation of the oral commissure, hypertrophy of the orbicularis oculi muscles, improvement of the gummy smile, and liplift.
- Although severe brow ptosis requires surgical intervention, mild ptosis or mild brow asymmetries can be corrected with carefully planned placement of neurotoxin injections.
- Neurotoxin injections cannot be considered a definitive treatment for necklift; however, mild platysmal banding can be treated to either delay open surgery or improve a less than perfect surgical result.
- Creative uses like the Nefertiti necklift can be used to replace or delay the need for an open procedure.

 A video accompanies this article, in which the senior author demonstrates injection areas for rejuvenation of the face—brow, eye, perioral, lip, and neck. Access the video, Cosmetic BoNTA for Minimally Invasive Facial Rejuvenation at: http://www.facialplastic.theclinics.com/

INTRODUCTION

Without question, the cosmetic use of botulinum toxin (BoNTA) has changed the practice of facial plastic surgery. Since its approval by the Food and Drug Administration in 2002 for treatment of glabellar frown lines, creative uses of the product have allowed surgeons to noninvasively shape the face. By understanding the underlying facial anatomy and the push-pull relationships of the muscles of facial expression, surgeons are now able to increase the muscular pull in one direction by eliminating the opposing force with neuromodulators.

The use of nonsurgical procedures is popular with today's patients because they can receive in-office treatments without taking time off from work. Some treatments with neurotoxins have become so effective that they have replaced traditional surgical procedures. This article present 5 of these procedures, which are off-label uses of neurotoxins.

CHEMICAL BROWLIFT

Facial rejuvenation of the upper third of the face has often focused on achieving the ideal brow contour and position. When analyzing the

Disclosures: T.C. Kontis: speaker's bureau for Allergan, Medicis, and Valeant.
[a] Department of Otolaryngology–Head and Neck Surgery, Johns Hopkins Medical Institutions, Baltimore, MD, USA; [b] Facial Plastic Surgicenter, LLC, 1838 Greene Tree Road, Suite 370, Baltimore, MD 21208, USA
* Corresponding author. Facial Plastic Surgicenter, LLC, 1838 Greene Tree Road, Suite 370, Baltimore, MD 21208, USA.
E-mail address: tckontis@aol.com

Facial Plast Surg Clin N Am 21 (2013) 285–298
http://dx.doi.org/10.1016/j.fsc.2013.02.009

aesthetics of the brow, the supraorbital rim and the upper eyelid crease are key factors to be taken into consideration. The ideal position of the female brow should be at the supraorbital rim medially, with the arc above the supraorbital rim laterally. The ideal male brow is described as positioned just above the supraorbital rim following a horizontal course along the rim. The ideal shape of the female brow is broad medially and tapering laterally, with its highest point at the lateral limbus or the lateral canthus according to individual preferences. The male brow is thicker and its shape does not taper. Lower brows are the product of aging and are often associated with feelings of sadness, grief, anger, and tiredness. Additionally, the position of the eyebrows can exacerbate the appearance of dermatochalasis of the upper eyelid.[1] Traditionally, forehead lifts have been used to rejuvenate the upper third of the face and improve brow position. More recently, neuromodulation of the brow depressors and elevators with BoNTA has been used to contour the brows to individual preference.

Surgical techniques available for the forehead include coronal, pretrichial, midforehead, direct and endoscopic approaches.[2] Traditional methods achieve brow repositioning by excising scalp skin and weakening of the muscular brow depressors. Endoscopic lifting often relies on skin redraping within the forehead and brow suspension. Since the introduction of the endoscopic browlift, it has gained rapid popularity due to its smaller incisions hidden in hair bearing surfaces. Browlifts are performed under general anesthesia and require 1 to 2 weeks of recovery. Although complications with forehead lifts are low, hematomas, seromas, alopecia, poor scarring, forehead dysesthesias, and injury to the frontal branch of the facial nerve are possible.[3]

A new alternative to the surgical approaches for brow rejuvenation has emerged with refinement in the use of BoNTA, in what is referred to as the *chemical browlift*.[4,5] The effects of BoNTA on the brow were initially noted as a side effect when treating hyperdynamic glabellar rhytides. Increased interbrow distance and medial brow elevation was an unintended consequence of treatment. Currently, BoNTA is used to intentionally achieve a browlift by selectively weakening brow depressors and allowing brow elevators to lift the brow. The frontalis muscle is responsible for brow elevation and its contraction results in horizontal rhytides along the forehead. Procerus, corrugator supercilii, and lateral orbicularis oculi are the main brow depressors. Inactivation of the depressor muscles permits the elevation of the brow by allowing the frontalis muscle to overcome its downward pull.

Procerus originates in the nasal bones and inserts on the lower forehead in skin between both brows acting as a brow depressor. Corrugator supercilii is also a medial depressor that originates in the superciliary arch and inserts into the skin of the medial brow and is primarily responsible for the vertical rhytides in the glabella. The lateral orbicularis oculi is responsible for lateral brow depression and so-called crow's feet rhytides. During a chemical browlift, medial elevation is mediated by weakening of corrugators and procerus muscles, and lateral elevation by weakening of the lateral orbicularis oculi muscles.

Treatment Goals in Browlift

A moderate browlift can be achieved by selectively weakening the brow depressors and allowing the frontalis to exert brow elevation.

Preoperative Planning

The injection sites medially and laterally are determined by examining the brow position during facial animation. Palpating the orbital rim prevents injection into the orbit that may lead to ptosis by affecting the levator palpebrae superioris. Having a patient frown and relax repetitively helps identify the length of the belly of the corrugator supercilii. Examining the area between the medial brows allows for identification of procerus muscles. Having a patient squint and smile demonstrates the crow's feet. When planning the injections, it is imperative to preserve muscle function in the forehead by not overly relaxing/treating the frontalis muscle with neurotoxin. If the frontalis muscle is not able to elevate the brow, brow ptosis may occur. It is important to notice that patients with severe brow ptosis are less likely to get a significant lift from a neurotoxin and might be better candidates for traditional or endoscopic browlifts.

Additional variations can be planned in cases where only certain portions of the brow are to be addressed or in cases of brow asymmetries. Frequently, some female patients request injections for contouring of the brow and elevation of the lateral brow only. In such cases, weakening the medial frontalis lowers the medial brow accentuating the lateral brow and providing the desired brow contour. Brow asymmetries where one brow is higher than the other can be addressed by attempting to lower the higher brow and raise the lower brow.

Procedural Approach

- Neurotoxin is placed into the procerus and corrugators muscles using approximately 5 to 7 injection sites.

- In addition, the lateral orbicularis muscle can be treated to increase the lateral lift.
- To treat the whole brow, a total of 20 to 25 BoNTA units (BU) or 60 to 75 abobotulinumtoxinA (Dysport) units (DU) may be necessary.

Note: The frontalis muscle superior to the brows should not be weakened, because it is the only mechanism to allow brow elevation.

Fig. 1 shows pretreatment and post-treatment results for a patient who underwent chemical browlift.

Potential Complications and Their Management

The treatment area is in close proximity to the muscles of the orbit and neurotoxin effect may spread to intraocular sites affecting the levator palpebrae superioris leading to ptosis. Care should be taken to keep the injection close to the surface of the skin to avoid deeper spread. Apraclonidine (Iodipine) 0.5% eyedrops are an α-adrenergic agonist used to correct this problem. By causing Müller muscle contraction, apraclonidine raises the eyelid margin by 1 to 2 mms.[6]

Not all patients obtain the same degree of brow elevation using this technique. Overtreatment of the frontalis muscle may negate any possible brow elevation achieved. The limitation of the degree of brow elevation is dictated by the unopposed action of frontalis muscle; after reaching the point of maximal weakening of brow depressors, further elevation requires surgical intervention.

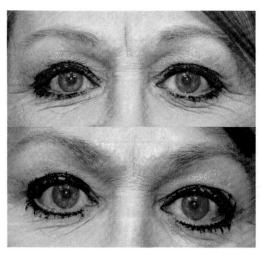

Fig. 1. Pretreatment (*top*) and post-treatment (*bottom*) photographs after BoNTA injection producing a chemical browlift.

Patients with severe brow ptosis are less likely to get a significant lift from a neurotoxin.

Immediate Postprocedural Care and Recovery

Post-treatment instructions are controversial. Although some physicians instruct their patients not to push on the injection sites, exercise, lay flat, or bend over for 4 hours, there are no data that show this prevents ptosis. Similarly, there are no studies that show movement of the injected muscles increases neurotoxin uptake.

Clinical Results in the Literature

Researchers have attempted to quantify the degree of brow elevation obtained by targeting different brow muscles. **Table 1** summarize the available literature on the effects of BoNTA treatment for brow elevation.

Studies examining the effect of treatment limited to the glabella only have shown that up to 3 mm of brow elevation can be achieved.[7,8] In 2007, Carruthers and Carruthers[8] published the largest series to date examining the effect of 20 BU to 40 BU to the glabella in 79 female patients. In their study, patients were examined every 2 weeks and maximum effect was seen at 12 weeks after injection, where up to 3 mm of brow elevation was seen in the lateral, central, and medial brow. In the study of treatment limited to the glabella, only 10 BU lead to medial brow ptosis. Different injection techniques have also achieved similar elevation. Huang and colleagues[9] reported on brow elevation after injection of 10 BU to the glabella and 10 BU superficially along the orbital rim with 4 evenly spaced injections, similar to the technique the authors describe, achieving up to 3 mm of brow elevation.

Studies that target the lateral orbicularis have also been published. Huilgol and colleagues[10] treated 7 patients by injecting 7 BU to 10 BU into the glabella and 0 BU to 2.5 BU to the lateral orbicularis, resulting in a 1 to 3 mm brow elevation in 5 of the 7 patients. Ahn and colleagues[11] treated the lateral orbicularis only at a dose of 10 BU and achieved an average of 4.83 mm of lateral brow elevation.

HYPERTROPHIC ORBICULARIS OCULI

Orbicularis oculi muscle hypertrophy is a condition that affects the lower eyelid and results in fullness when smiling or squinting, producing a tired look at rest.

The orbicularis oculi muscle surrounds the eye and is divided into 3 parts: orbital, preseptal, and pretarsal. The primary function of pretarsal muscle

Table 1
Summary of references articles of brow elevation obtained with botulinum toxin injection

Article	Study Type	Patient Population	Injection Site and Dose	Timeframe	Results
Huilgol et al,[10] 1999	Prospective case series	7 Patients	7–10 BU to glabella and 0–2.5 BU to lateral orbicularis oculi	1 mo	1–3 mm of Brow elevation in 5 of 7 patients
Frankel,[7] 1999	Prospective case series	30 Patients	20 BU to glabella	2 wk	32% Had an increase in medial brow and 48% in the central brow
Huang et al,[9] 2000	Case series	11 Patients	10 BU to glabella and 10 BU superficially along the superior orbital rim	7–10 d	Average 2–3 mm elevation
Ahn et al,[11] 2000	Prospective case series	22 Patients	10 BU to lateral orbicularis oculi	2 wk	Average elevation of 1 mm at midpupillary line and 4.83 mm at the lateral canthus
Carruthers and Carruthers,[8] 2007	Retrospective case series	79 Patients	20–40 BU to glabella	Every 2 wk for 20 wk	Central, medial, and lateral elevation peaked at wk 12 with up to 3 mm of elevation

is involuntary closing of the eye. Hypertrophy of the muscle in this region may cause bunching of the skin, infraorbital rhytides, and narrowing of the palpebral aperture during contraction. Fullness in the pretarsal portion is different from fullness in the preseptal portion of the eye. Although often overlooked, pretarsal fullness is due to muscular hypertrophy, whereas preseptal fullness is due to the more traditional concept of orbital fat prominence.[12,13] To treat orbicularis oculi hypertrophy during lower eyelid blepharoplasty, a subciliary incision is necessary to allow for resection of a strip of the hypertrophic muscle at the pretarsal region.[14] The risk of this approach is scar contraction with lower eyelid retraction, eyelid malposition, scleral show, and ectropion. Although eyelid retraction after lower eyelid blepharoplasty is an infrequent complication, it is feared given that correction is difficult.[15]

Hypertrophy of the orbicularis oculi can now be addressed with BoNTA.[16] The lower eyelid can be treated with neurotoxin to improve fullness and flatten the appearance of the eyelid. Additionally, benefits of treating the lower eyelid include decreasing rhytides and widening of the palpebral aperture, which is considered more attractive.[17,18] These effects become more pronounced when the crow's feet region is concomitantly treated.

Treatment Goals in Hypertrophic Orbicularis Oculi

Hypertrophy of the orbicularis oculi muscle can cause a fullness of the lower eyelid when smiling or squinting. By weakening the muscle with neurotoxin, flattening of the lower eyelid roll is achieved.

Preoperative Planning

Accurate diagnosis is key in these patients who complain of lower eyelid bags. Patients must be counseled on the differences between lower lid fat herniation and orbicularis muscle hypertrophy and treated appropriately. Check for ectropion and dry-eye or Sjögren symptoms before injections because weakening of the orbicularis may exacerbate these conditions. The tone and elasticity of the lower eyelid should be evaluated before injection by performing a snap test.

Procedural Approach

- BoNTA (1–2 BU or 3–6 DU) is injected at the midpupillary line approximately 3 mm below the lash line.
- A single injection is placed per eyelid.
- The injection is immediately subcutaneous.

Note: Because of the increased zone of effect for Dysport, BoNTA may be preferred for these injections.

Fig. 2 shows pretreatment and post-treatment results for a patient smiling before and after neurotoxin injection to the lower eyelid roll.

Potential Complications and Their Management

Widening of the palpebral aperture may result in dry eyes and disturb normal blinking. Inject with caution in patients with lax lower eyelids or with dry eye syndrome. Bruising may occur after injection.

Immediate postprocedural care

No specific care is necessary immediately after treatment. Cold compresses may be applied for comfort or possible mild bruising. Patients may return to regular activities immediately after injection.

Clinical Results in the Literature

The first report of BoNTA to the lower eyelid was published in 2001 by Flynn and colleagues,[18] describing direct injections of 2 BU in the lower eyelid for infraorbital rhytides. In addition to the effect on the rhytides, there was an increase in the palpebral aperture in 40% of patients. This increase was seen as a favorable cosmetic change. The effect in the palpebral aperture was accentuated

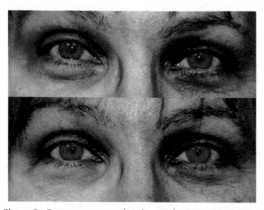

Fig. 2. Pretreatment (*top*) and post-treatment (*bottom*) photographs after BoNTA injection to the lower eyelid for hypertrophy of orbicularis oculi muscles seen when the patient smiles.

when the crow's feet were treated at the same time achieving an increase of 1.3 mm at rest and 3 mm when smiling. The investigators comment that the results were more notable in Asian patients. Subsequently, the same group conducted a study to evaluate the effect of different doses to the lower eyelid ranging from 1 BU to 8 BU. Increasing doses progressively widened the palpebral aperture; however, an unacceptable rate of side effects was encountered at higher doses. When 2 BU were used per eyelid, no patients experienced any side effects, whereas more than half of the patients had problems with incomplete sphincter function and edema at 8 BU doses.[17]

REJUVENATION OF ORAL COMMISSURE

Downward turn of the oral commissure is a sign of an aging mouth that gives an appearance of being tired, sad, or even bitter. The lateral oral commissure can extend, forming a groove, and contribute to the marionette appearance. In severe cases, particularly in older patients, it can be a site for drooling and angular cheilitis may develop. This area can represent a problem even after successful rejuvenation with facelift. During facelift, correction of the corner of the mouth would require excessive pulling that would result in a fishmouth deformity, an unnatural and obviously operated look. Although patients can be bothered by this appearance, improvement of the corner of the mouth can be achieved by treating the oral commissure.

Commissuroplasty

Traditionally, a commissuroplasty or lift of the oral commissure has been the procedure used to address this area. The technique involves a full thickness excision of skin superiorly and laterally to the oral commissure to elevate the corner of the mouth while camouflaging the incision parallel and immediately outside to the vermilion border.[19,20] As a result of the procedure, a visible scar is created. Although most patients find the incision not noticeable and easily concealed, hypertophic scarring is always a possibility. Another potential disadvantage of commissuroplasty is overcorrection of the lift where the commissures are turned upwards, creating an unnatural look often referred to as a *joker appearance*.

Filler and Neurotoxin

Presently, commissuroplasty has been replaced by augmentation filling to efface the oral commissure groove and neurotoxin injection to the depressor anguli oris (DAO).[21–23] Neurotoxin alone can be used in this area but most often must be combined with filler injections to the oral commissure. The DAO is a facial muscle that originates in the outer surface of the mandible at the oblique line of the mandible and inserts into the modiolus at the angle of the mouth. Its function is to depress and lateralize the lips and, together with the mandibular ligament, form the mentolabial groove. Direct injection into the DAO with BoNTA allows for weakening of the muscle and results in elevation of the corner of the lips by action of the levator anguli oris and the zygomaticus major and minor muscles. DAO injection is an outpatient procedure that allows patients to return to their regular activities immediately after injection. The risks of permanent scarring are avoided, although it does require repeat injection.

Treatment Goals of Oral Commissure Neuromodulation

The main objective of neuromodulation of the DAO is lip rejuvenation by lifting the downward turn of the corner of the lip.

Preoperative Planning

Careful assessment of the perioral muscles should always be done at rest and with contraction. The DAO muscle may be palpated while having patients actively frown from the origin in the mandible to its insertion into the corner of the mouth. Patients should be appropriately counseled that DAO injection does not improve severely depressed oral commissures, which most likely require filler injection in addition to DAO injection, and does not elevate the marionette lines.

Procedural Approach

- A single injection per muscle is suggested and well tolerated.
- The DAO muscle should be palpated while having patients actively frown. If the belly of the muscle cannot be palpated, an approximate estimate of its location can be made by going 1 cm lateral to the oral commissure and then 1 cm inferiorly.
- Inject approximately 2–5 BU (or 6–15 DU) deeply into each muscle.
- Alternatively, to avoid other perioral muscles, injections may be placed into the muscle along the mandibular border.

Fig. 3 shows pretreatment and post-treatment photographs.

Potential Complications and Their Management

Overtreatment of this area can lead to oral incompetence. Using conservative doses of BoNTA, it is

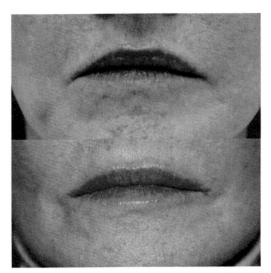

Fig. 3. Pretreatment (*top*) and post-treatment (*bottom*) photographs after BoNTA injection to the DAO combined with filler injection at the lateral oral commissures to elevate the corners of the mouth.

more likely that only a mild improvement in the downturned oral commissure is seen, especially in patients with heavy surrounding skin. The major risk of BoNTA is diffusion of the product to perioral muscles, which may affect the smile or expression.

Immediate Postprocedural Care

No specific care is necessary post-treatment and bruising is unlikely. Patients may return to regular activities immediately after injection.

Clinical Results in the Literature

Treatment by chemical neuromodulation of the DAO to improve the downward turn of the oral commissure is increasingly described in the literature, making evident a trend favoring this technique over open commissuroplasty.[21,22,24] Investigators emphasize injection technique and understanding of the facial musculature around the oral commissure as critical in adequately identifying the DAO to achieve corner of the mouth elevation without affecting the other muscles involved in lip movement. Injection along the mandibular border is recommended to avoid perioral muscles. Available publications do not report problems with asymmetric smile after meticulous injection techniques. Predictable and replicable results are shown with few risks and minimal discomfort. The degree of elevation has not been objectively quantified in the literature.

GUMMY SMILE

The smile is a facial expression that transmits happiness and is fundamental to sociability and human connection. Excessive gingival display above the dentate line when smiling is referred in the literature as *gummy smile* or even a *horse smile*. Patients with gummy smiles are often self-conscious and restrain themselves from a full smile, often seeking consultation for possible intervention.

Evaluation of this problem includes examining the dynamic contribution of the maxilla, the gingiva, and the lips. Excessive vertical height can affect the position of the lips, which may be addressed with orthognathic surgery, such as a Le Fort type I osteotomy.[25,26] Delayed teeth eruption is an abnormality in which the gingiva covers the dental crown, allowing aesthetic crown lengthening as a possible intervention.[27] Commonly, hyperfunction of the lip elevators muscles with excessive lip retraction or short lips can also be the cause of this problem.

Levator labii superioris (LLS), LLS alaeque nasi (LLSAN), levator anguli oris, zygomaticus muscles, and risorius are the facial muscles involved in lip elevation. Depressor septi nasi muscle can also contribute to elevation of the lip at the midline.[28] LLS, LLSAN, and zygomaticus minor provide vertical elevation whereas levator anguli oris, zygomaticus major, and risorius also contribute to oral commissure elevation.

Lip-lengthening procedures that reposition and lengthen the upper lip have traditionally been used to address excessive gingival show during smile.[29–32] The lip is approached transorally and an ellipse excision of the mucosa in the gingival labial sulcus is performed, allowing for inferior repositioning and lengthening of the lip on closure. For additional lengthening, myotomies at the insertion of the lip elevator muscles can be performed through this incision. The main muscle targeted is the LLS, allowing for sparring of the oral commissure. The muscles can be divided through this approach without disrupting the orbicularis oris.[31,32] The LLS originates along the orbital rim in the maxilla and inserts into the skin lateral to the nostril and on the upper lip, blending with the orbicularis oris. Lip lengthening can be used for cases of hyperfunctional lip elevation, short lips, or even in cases of excessive maxillary height when patients decline orthognathic surgery. The procedure can be performed under local anesthesia in the office setting. Potential complication with wound healing as well as transient lip numbness can result from this procedure. More recently, BoNTA injection to lower the upper lip, in order to minimize gingival show, has emerged as an alternative treatment option.[33] Techniques aimed at reducing gingival show target the LLSAN muscles.[34] The injection is well tolerated and an outpatient patient procedure that allows patients to return to their regular activities immediately after injection.

Treatment Goals in Correcting Gummy Smile

The main objective during this injection is to decrease gingival display during smile by injecting the lip elevators.

Preoperative Planning

Evaluation during smiling allows examination of the exposed gingiva. As discussed previously, evaluation of this problem includes examining the dynamic contribution of the maxilla, the gingiva, and the lips. Patients with excessive maxillary vertical height or with delayed teeth eruption should be appropriately counseled and referred to an oromaxillary specialist.

Procedural Approach

- A single injection per side is suggested and well tolerated.
- The LLSAN muscle is targeted by injecting 3 mm to 5 mm lateral to the nostril.
- Inject approximately 2–4 BU or 6–12 DU deeply to achieve muscular injection.

Pretreatment and post-treatment photographs are shown in **Fig. 4.**

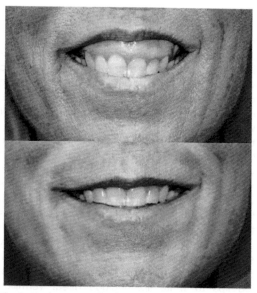

Fig. 4. Pretreatment (*top*) and post-treatment (*bottom*) photographs after BoNTA injection for treatment of a gummy smile.

Potential Complications and Their Management

The major risk is that BoNTA may affect the wrong perioral muscles and affect the smile or expression. Injecting into the lateral corner of the mouth can lead to oral incompetence.

Immediate Postprocedural Care

There are no post-treatment instructions and patients may return to regular activities immediately after injection. Bruising in this area is unlikely; however, care must be taken to stay lateral to avoid the angular artery.

Clinical Results in the Literature

Treatment of excessive gingival show by neuromodulation of the lip elevators has been increasingly reported in the literature. Sucupira and Abramovitz[33] published a case series evaluating 52 patients who underwent injection for treatment of gummy smile and photo documented response after injection. In the study, gingival display decreased from an average of 3.6 mm to 0.58 mm with an increase in lip length from 12.48 mm to 19 mm. Average patient satisfaction was extremely high, at 9.75, from a 10-point scale, and up to 94% of the patients stated they would repeat the injection. Similar results were shown by Polo[35] in a case series of 30 patients, which observed a decreased gingival show from 5.2 mm to 0.09 mm and a lip drop of 5.1 mm. No complications were reported in either study.

LIPLIFT

Full lips provide a youthful and beautiful appearance, whereas thin lips are often perceived as less attractive and a sign of aging. Increasing vermilion height, improving the definition of lip contour, and increasing the overall fullness of the lip is increasingly a desired feature in women for which cosmetic consultation is sought. During the aging process, the ratio of the red lips to white lips is altered with reduction in the height of vermilion border and an increase in the dermal area of the upper lip in a condition described as vermilion lip hypoplasia.[36] Vertical wrinkles and loss of Cupid's bow are other undesired changes that become evident in the aging lips.

Techniques to reshape the lip are increasingly sought in cosmetic surgery and facial rejuvenation. Surgical options available to increase the ratio of red lips to white lips include direct vermilion advancements, subnasal liplift, and V-Y advancements.[20,37,38] Direct vermilion advancements involve excision of the skin immediately above the vermilion border with advancement of the red lip superiorly. Subnasal liplift increases the red lip through direct excision of skin under the nasal vestibule of the nose. Intraoral V-Y advancements can be designed to increase lip projection. Because of external scarring, perioral rejuvenation did not receive much attention in the past. More recently, the use of soft tissue augmentation with filler technology that avoids scarring while restoring volume has gained increasing popularity. Injectable hyaluronic acid can improve the definition of the vermilion border, improve lip contour, and increase the red-to-white lip ratio.[39] Although volume restoration has traditionally been the rejuvenating approach for the lips, a combination of fillers and BoNTA has emerged as an available strategy. Treatment of the perioral region with BoNTA injections in the orbicularis oris can complement other rejuvenation strategies.[39,40] The orbicularis oris muscle is a circular muscle that functions as a sphincter that surrounds the mouth. The deep fibers bring the lips together, whereas the more superficial fibers pucker the lips forward. The muscle fibers are naturally aligned so as to pull toward the center. Weakening this pull allows the upper lip elevators and the lower lip depressors to increase their displacement of the lips. The end result is a more visible pink lip with slight lip eversion. This technique produces a small augmentation in the lips, a possible 1 mm to 2 mm increase in pink lip visibility. Patients should not expect the same results as fillers, but this procedure can be used in addition to fillers in patients with very thin lips. Additionally, fine vertical perioral rhytides, often referred to as *lipstick lines* or *smokers' lines*, are improved as a result of these injections.

Treatment Goals in Liplift

A small improvement in the visible pink lip can be achieved by the use of neurotoxins. This can be used to enhance the upper and/or lower lips.

Preoperative Planning

The lips and the perioral muscles should be evaluated. Articulation of the letters E and O are of particular assistance. Careful patient selection avoids this technique in patients who depend on their perioral muscles, such as singers and wind instrument musicians. **Fig. 5** shows pretreatment and post-treatment results.

Procedural Approach

- BoNTA is injected at the base of the philtrum at the vermillion border.

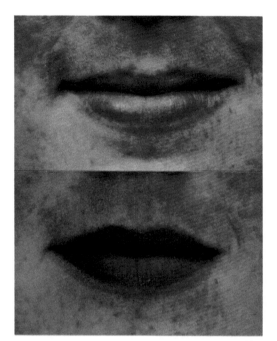

Fig. 5. Pretreatment (*top*) and post-treatment (*bottom*) photographs after BoNTA injection to produce a chemical liplift.

- Injections are superficial and symmetry is key.
- Both upper and lower lips can be injected.
- Two injection sites per lip, with one injection in each lip quadrant is recommended.
- The corresponding location of the lower lip can also be injected.
- Approximately 1–2 BU (or 3–6 DU) is used for each injection.

Note: Careful attention should be made to avoid the medial portion of the lip over Cupid's bow and the corners of the lips.

Potential Complications and Their Management

Asymmetry of the lips can be reduced by insuring the injections are placed precisely and symmetrically. Injection at the midline should be avoided because it can lead to flattening of Cupid's bow. When the corners of lips are avoided, weakness in the muscles that elevate the lips is prevented, thereby preventing difficulties with oral competence, drooling, and speech.

Immediate Postprocedural Care

This is a sensitive area and cold compresses may be applied for comfort. Patients may return to regular activities immediately after injection.

Clinical Results in the Literature

The literature continues to describe expansion of the use of BoNTA to include the lower third of the face and the lips. Volume loss continues to be the main paradigm of improving lip aging and cosmesis. The additional benefits of complementary intervention with neuromodulation, however, are becoming increasingly evident. A recent prospective randomized trial by Carruthers and colleagues[41] emphasized these advantages in perioral and lower face rejuvenation by demonstrating better and longer-lasting results when combining BoNTA with fillers. In their study, 90 female patients were randomized to filler alone, BoNTA alone, or a combination of both. BoNTA injection was not limited to orbicularis but also included DAO and mentalis. Combination treatment provided the best perioral rejuvenation and lip fullness over either intervention alone as judged by blinded reviewers. Additionally, combination treatment prolonged the duration of the effects achieved potentially by minimizing facial contraction and allowing the filler to remain in place.

PLATYSMAL BANDING

The platysma muscle is a thin superficial muscle that originates on the clavicle and upper chest and inserts onto the superficial muscular aponeurotic system, the skin of the lower face, the facial muscles, and the mandible. Although in youth it is a continuous sheet, in the elderly, the muscle may splay centrally and produce prominent vertical bands. Accentuation of these vertical fibrous platysma bands and herniation of underlying fat pads as the muscle separates, most commonly at their anterior edges, is characteristic of the aging neck. Platysmal bands can be prominent in patients with thin necks, thin skin, and patients without abundant overlying fat. Rhytidectomy has remained the main treatment option. Plication of the medial platysmal bands and lateral suspension of the posterior borders can help address their appearance. Corset plastymaplasty with submental suspension after midline fat removal reinforces the muscle sling and is advocated to prevent recurrent banding.[42] Despite the success obtained with these procedures, residual or recurrent banding remains a challenge.[43]

Rejuvenation of the aging neck with BoNTA treatment of platysmal banding has emerged as a safe and minimally invasive approach.[44–47] This technique is ideal for younger patients in their mid-30s or early 40s with good skin elasticity and for patients who already underwent facelift and have residual or recurrent banding.

Recuperation is minimal after injection of the platysmal bands. Patients with particularly heavy and hard necks might not experience the desired results. Appropriate surgical candidates should be given the option for lower face and necklift surgery.

Treatment Goals in Vertical Platysma Banding

Softening of vertical platysma banding with direct neurotoxin injection is a tool in neck rejuvenation.

Preoperative Planning

Vertical platysmal bands in the neck that are seen at rest are accentuated with neck tightening and forced jaw opening. Having patients grimace and tighten the neck to accentuate the bands and identify the problem muscles makes injection easier to perform.

Procedural Approach

- With the platysma muscle in full contraction, the edge of the muscle band is grasped with 2 fingers while the muscle is injected.
- The needle is placed deeply into the muscle, between the operator's fingers and perpendicular to the muscle fibers.
- Approximately 3–5 BU (or 6–25 DU) is injected into each injection site, for a total of 15–20 BU (or 45–60 DU) per band.
- A series of approximately 3 injections is placed down the length of the band approximately 1.5 cm to 2 cm apart.
- If lateral bands are prominent on full contraction, then these can be injected in the same fashion, although they often need fewer units.
- Begin injections at the cervicomental angle and work inferiorly, staying approximately 2 cm to 2.5 cm below the mandibular border

so as not to affect the upper facial muscles of expression.

Fig. 6 shows the results from BoNTA treatment to mild platysmal bands.

Potential Complications and Their Management

Overinjection in this region may affect the deeper musculature resulting in dysphagia or dysphonia.[48] Bruising is not uncommon and has been reported in as high as 20% of patients.[45] Patients with heavy necks may not be good candidates for this procedure because the results of injection may not be impressive.

Immediate Postprocedural Care

Hold pressure to prevent bruising. Patients may return to regular activities immediately.

Clinical Results in the Literature

The case series available in the literature have reported high success rates and satisfaction with the use of BoNTA in platysmal bands. The dose used in the bands has varied between studies. Matarasso and colleagues[44] published their experience in 1500 patients, where 50 to 100 BU were used per band, with a maximum of 250 BU per patient. In this study, reported complications included neck discomfort in 10% of patients, 1 patient with neck weakness, and 1 patient with dysphagia. Subsequently Kane[23] published experience with platysmal banding treatment at significantly lower doses. In that study, 44 patients were treated with a maximal dose of 40 BU per patient and 7.5 BU to 12.5 BU per band without any dysphagia or dysphonia.

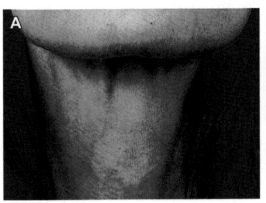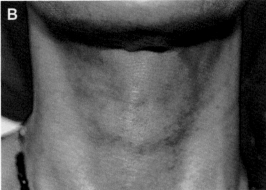

Fig. 6. (A) Before and (B) after treatment of the platysmal bands with BoNTA.

THE NEFERTITI NECKLIFT

The ancient Egyptian queen, Nefertiti, was once referred to as the most beautiful woman in the world. The hand-painted limestone bust of Nefertiti is one of the most copied images in ancient Egypt, and currently forms part of the collection of Neues Museum in Berlin. This famous art piece depicts an elegant beautiful woman with a sculpted jawline.

Loss of jawline definition occurs with aging, because skin elasticity and volume progressively decline. Facelift has been the surgical technique traditionally used to improve mandibular contour. The results obtained with the Nefertiti necklift have been compared with the results obtained with a minilift, which is often used in younger patients in whom less dissection is required for neck rejuvenation.[49]

Most techniques that use BoNTA to rejuvenate the neck have concentrated on treating platysma bands, whereas the Nefertiti technique uses BoNTA to emphasize definition of the mandible.[50] The injections target the platysma muscle at the level of the mandible. The platysma muscle is a neck depressor that originates at the clavicle and fascia of the upper chest and inserts onto the mandible and skin of the chin and cheek. Weakening of the muscle allows facial elevators to elevate the sagging skin over the lower face and more clearly define the mandibular border, achieving a slim and smooth jawline with a well-defined cervicomental angle.

Treatment Goals with the Nefertiti Necklift

Improve jawline definition to achieve neck rejuvenation.

Preoperative Planning

Patient selection is extremely important when performing this procedure. Patients who desire a more defined mandibular contour should be assessed for the extent of platysma pull on their lower face. It is suggested that patients be asked to contract the platysma muscles and, if the mandibular border becomes less visible, they are a good candidate for this procedure.

Procedural Approach

- Injections of BoNTA are placed along the inferior aspect of the mandible and in the upper aspect of the strongest lateral platysma band.
- Injections are deep into the muscle.
- Approximately 15–20 BU (45–60 DU) are used per side in equal amounts.
- Sites lateral to the nasolabial fold are preferred for injection to avoid weakening the depressor labii inferioris muscle.

Fig. 7 reveals the results that may be seen in patients who are good candidates for this procedure.

Potential Complications and Management

Extending these injections too far medially can affect the depressor labii inferioris and cause an asymmetric smile. Do not inject medial to a line drawn down from the nasolabial fold to the mandible. Overinjection of this area can also result in dysphagia if the deeper neck muscles are affected. Excessive pull upwards on the lower face can result in irregular bunching of the tissue over the mandible.

Immediate Postprocedural Care

Hold pressure to prevent bruising. The recovery for the Nefertiti necklift is immediate. Minilifts are often chosen by patients because of the decreased downtime in comparison with traditional facelifts, given their more limited dissection. The Nefertiti

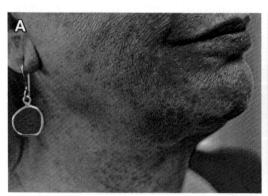 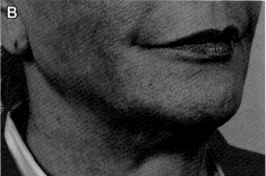

Fig. 7. (*A*) Before and (*B*) after Nefertiti necklift neurotoxin injection procedure.

Table 2
Summary of procedures described with targeted muscles, botulinum toxin doses, and injection sites

Procedure	Targeted Muscles	Units	Injection Site
Chemical browlift	Procerus, corrugator supercili, and orbicularis oculi	20–25 BU (60–75 DU) total	Injection sites targeting the glabellar complex and lateral orbicularis
Hypertrophic orbicularis oculi	Lower eyelid orbicularis oculi	1–2 BU (3–6 DU) per eyelid	Single injection 3 mm below lash line at the midpupillary line
Oral commissure lift	DAO	2–5 BU (6–15 DU) per side	Single injection 1 cm lateral and inferior to oral commissure
Gummy smile	Levator labii superior aleque nasai	2–4 BU (6–12 DU) per side	Single injection 3–5 mm lateral to the nostril
Liplift	Orbicularis oris	2–4 BU (6–12 DU) total	Symmetric injections on the left and right sides of the vermillion border avoiding Cupid's bow
Platysmal banding	Platysma	15–20 BU (45–60 DU) per band	Series on injections into the band starting at the cervicomental angle placed 1–2 cm apart
Nefertiti necklift	Platysma	15–20 BU (45–60 DU) per side	Series of injections to the platysma along the inferior border of the mandible and lateral to the nasolabial fold

necklift provides an option where no downtime is necessary and is appealing to patients.

Clinical Results in the Literature

Levy first described the Nefertiti technique in 2007 by treating 120 patients with injections along the mandible with 15 BU to 20 BU per neck side. During follow-up at 2 weeks, noticeable contouring and elevation of the jawline were seen. Side effects included dysphagia in 2 patients, irregular elevation in 2 patients, and smile asymmetry in another 2 patients that resolved with time.[50] Further cosmetic mandibular contouring with BoNTA can be achieved by injecting the masseter muscle. By weakening the masseteric muscle, the muscle bulk is decreased and a slimmer facial contour is created. Kim and colleagues[51] published a retrospective case series on 1021 patients with such injections, describing aesthetically pleasing results.

SUMMARY

Selected facial cosmetic surgical procedures have become obsolete with the creative use of BoNTA. Mild brow ptosis can be treated with neurotoxin before patients must resort to a surgical procedure. Similarly, for patients who have mild platysmal banding or recurrent banding postoperatively, neurotoxin injection can improve the band tension. In patients with severe banding, BoNTA injection is not an alternative to surgery. In the authors' practice, however, neurotoxin has replaced the need for orbicularis resection of the lower lid for muscle hypertrophy, commissureplasty for ptotic oral commissures, lip advancement surgeries for small upper lips, and lip lengthening procedures for patients with a gummy smile. In selected patients, the authors are able to better define the neckline with neurotoxins by performing a Nefertiti necklift. **Table 2** summarizes the procedures described for BoNTA treatment to these areas. As newer products are developed and physicians continue to explore less invasive procedures, the authors predict more noninvasive techniques will become the mainstay for facial rejuvenation.

SUPPLEMENTARY DATA

Supplementary data related to this article can be found online at http://dx.doi.org/10.1016/j.fsc.2013.02.009.

REFERENCES

1. Angelos PC, Stallworth CL, Wang TD. Forehead lifting: state of the art. Facial Plast Surg 2011; 27(1):50–7.

2. Puig CM, LaFerriere KA. A retrospective comparison of open and endoscopic brow-lifts. Arch Facial Plast Surg 2002;4(4):221–5.

3. Graham DW, Heller J, Kurkjian TJ, et al. Brow lift in facial rejuvenation: a systematic literature review of open versus endoscopic techniques. Plast Reconstr Surg 2011;128(4):335e–41e.

4. Frankel AS, Kamer FM. Chemical brow lift. Arch Otolaryngol Head Neck Surg 1998;124:321–3.

5. Chen AH, Frankel AS. Altering brow contour with botulinum toxin. Facial Plast Surg Clin North Am 2003;11(4):457–64.

6. Matarasso SL. Complications of botulinum A exotoxin for hyperfunctional lines. Dermatol Surg 1998;24(11):1249–54.

7. Frankel AS. Botox for rejuvenation of the periorbital region. Facial Plast Surg 1999;15(3):255–62.

8. Carruthers A, Carruthers J. Eyebrow height after botulinum toxin type A to the glabella. Dermatol Surg 2007;33(Spec No 1):S26–31.

9. Huang W, Rogachefsky AS, Foster JA. Browlift with botulinum toxin. Dermatol Surg 2000;26(1):55–60.

10. Huilgol SC, Carruthers A, Carruthers JD. Raising eyebrows with botulinum toxin. Dermatol Surg 1999;25(5):373–5 [discussion: 6].

11. Ahn MS, Catten M, Maas CS. Temporal brow lift using botulinum toxin A. Plast Reconstr Surg 2000; 105(3):1129–35 [discussion: 36–9].

12. Furnas DW. Festoons of orbicularis muscle as a cause of baggy eyelids. Plast Reconstr Surg 1978;61(4):540–6.

13. Loeb R. Necessity for partial resection of the orbicularis oculi muscle in blepharoplasties in some young patients. Plast Reconstr Surg 1977;60(2): 176–8.

14. Bernardi C, Dura S, Amata PL. Treatment of orbicularis oculi muscle hypertrophy in lower lid blepharoplasty. Aesthetic Plast Surg 1998;22(5):349–51.

15. Manku K, Leong JK, Ghabrial R. Cicatricial ectropion: repair with myocutaneous flaps and canthopexy. Clin Experiment Ophthalmol 2006;34(7):677–81.

16. Raspaldo H, Baspeyras M, Bellity P, et al. Upper- and mid-face anti-aging treatment and prevention using onabotulinumtoxin A: the 2010 multidisciplinary French consensus—part 1. J Cosmet Dermatol 2011;10(1):36–50.

17. Flynn TC, Carruthers JA, Carruthers JA, et al. Botulinum A toxin (BOTOX) in the lower eyelid: dose-finding study. Dermatol Surg 2003;29(9):943–50 [discussion: 50–1].

18. Flynn TC, Carruthers JA, Carruthers JA. Botulinum-A toxin treatment of the lower eyelid improves infraorbital rhytides and widens the eye. Dermatol Surg 2001;27(8):703–8.

19. Perkins SW. The corner of the mouth lift and management of the oral commissure grooves. Facial Plast Surg Clin North Am 2007;15(4):471–6, vii.

20. Weston GW, Poindexter BD, Sigal RK, et al. Lifting lips: 28 years of experience using the direct excision approach to rejuvenating the aging mouth. Aesthet Surg J 2009;29(2):83–6.

21. Goldman A, Wollina U. Elevation of the corner of the mouth using botulinum toxin type a. J Cutan Aesthet Surg 2010;3(3):145–50.

22. Carruthers J, Carruthers A. BOTOX use in the mid and lower face and neck. Semin Cutan Med Surg 2001;20(2):85–92.

23. Kane MA. The functional anatomy of the lower face as it applies to rejuvenation via chemodenervation. Facial Plast Surg 2005;21(1):55–64.

24. Le Louarn C, Buis J, Buthiau D. Treatment of depressor anguli oris weakening with the face recurve concept. Aesthet Surg J 2006;26(5):603–11.

25. Ezquerra F, Berrazueta MJ, Ruiz-Capillas A, et al. New approach to the gummy smile. Plast Reconstr Surg 1999;104(4):1143–50 [discussion: 51–2].

26. Fowler P. Orthodontics and orthognathic surgery in the combined treatment of an excessively "gummy smile". N Z Dent J 1999;95(420):53–4.

27. Allen EP. Surgical crown lengthening for function and esthetics. Dent Clin North Am 1993;37(2):163–79.

28. McAlister RW, Harkness EM, Nicoll JJ. An ultrasound investigation of the lip levator musculature. Eur J Orthod 1998;20(6):713–20.

29. Litton C, Fournier P. Simple surgical correction of the gummy smile. Plast Reconstr Surg 1979;63(3): 372–3.

30. Rubinstein A, Kostianovsky A. Cosmetic surgery for the malformation of the laugh: original technique. Prensa Med Argent 1973;60:952.

31. Miskinyar SA. A new method for correcting a gummy smile. Plast Reconstr Surg 1983;72(3):397–400.

32. Ishida LH, Ishida LC, Ishida J, et al. Myotomy of the levator labii superioris muscle and lip repositioning: a combined approach for the correction of gummy smile. Plast Reconstr Surg 2010;126(3):1014–9.

33. Sucupira E, Abramovitz A. A simplified method for smile enhancement: botulinum toxin injection for gummy smile. Plast Reconstr Surg 2012;130(3):726–8.

34. Hwang WS, Hur MS, Hu KS, et al. Surface anatomy of the lip elevator muscles for the treatment of gummy smile using botulinum toxin. Angle Orthod 2009;79(1):70–7.

35. Polo M. Botulinum toxin type A (Botox) for the neuromuscular correction of excessive gingival display on smiling (gummy smile). Am J Orthod Dentofacial Orthop 2008;133(2):195–203.

36. Penna V, Stark GB, Eisenhardt SU, et al. The aging lip: a comparative histological analysis of age-related changes in the upper lip complex. Plast Reconstr Surg 2009;124(2):624–8.

37. Holden PK, Sufyan AS, Perkins SW. Long-term analysis of surgical correction of the senile upper lip. Arch Facial Plast Surg 2011;13(5):332–6.

38. Jacono AA, Quatela VC. Quantitative analysis of lip appearance after V-Y lip augmentation. Arch Facial Plast Surg 2004;6(3):172–7.

39. Jacono AA. A new classification of lip zones to customize injectable lip augmentation. Arch Facial Plast Surg 2008;10(1):25–9.

40. Raspaldo H, Niforos FR, Gassia V, et al. Lower-face and neck antiaging treatment and prevention using onabotulinumtoxin A: the 2010 multidisciplinary French consensus—part 2. J Cosmet Dermatol 2011;10(2):131–49.

41. Carruthers J, Carruthers A, Monheit GD, et al. Multicenter, randomized, parallel-group study of onabotulinumtoxinA and hyaluronic acid dermal fillers (24-mg/ml smooth, cohesive gel) alone and in combination for lower facial rejuvenation: satisfaction and patient-reported outcomes. Dermatol Surg 2010;36(Suppl 4):2135–45.

42. Jacob CI, Kaminer MS. The corset platysma repair: a technique revisited. Dermatol Surg 2002;28(3): 257–62.

43. Owsley JQ. Face lifting: problems, solutions, and an outcome study. Plast Reconstr Surg 2000;105(1): 302–13 [discussion: 314–5].

44. Matarasso A, Matarasso SL, Brandt FS, et al. Botulinum A exotoxin for the management of platysma bands. Plast Reconstr Surg 1999;103(2):645–52 [discussion: 53–5].

45. Matarasso A, Matarasso SL. Botulinum A exotoxin for the management of platysma bands. Plast Reconstr Surg 2003;112(Suppl 5):138S–40S.

46. Kane MA. Nonsurgical treatment of platysma bands with injection of botulinum toxin a revisited. Plast Reconstr Surg 2003;112(Suppl 5):125S–6S.

47. Brandt FS, Boker A. Botulinum toxin for the treatment of neck lines and neck bands. Dermatol Clin 2004; 22(2):159–66.

48. Carruthers J, Carruthers A. Practical cosmetic Botox techniques. J Cutan Med Surg 1999;3(Suppl 4): S49–52.

49. Rousso DE, Brys AK. Minimal incision face-lifting. Facial Plast Surg 2012;28(1):76–88.

50. Levy PM. The 'Nefertiti lift': a new technique for specific re-contouring of the jawline. J Cosmet Laser Ther 2007;9(4):249–52.

51. Kim NH, Chung JH, Park RH, et al. The use of botulinum toxin type A in aesthetic mandibular contouring. Plast Reconstr Surg 2005;115(3):919–30.

Autologous Cell Therapy
Will It Replace Dermal Fillers?

Robert A. Weiss, MD[a,b,]*

KEYWORDS

- Autologous cell therapy • Autologous fibroblasts • Wrinkle correction • Aging face
- Facial rejuvenation

KEY POINTS

- Unlike conventional fillers, cultured autologous fibroblast cells are injected more superficially and may require months to show improvement.
- This treatment offers the promise of sustained growth of living cells, which may have greater persistence than other fillers.
- Fibroblasts are not a volume filler, and fibroblast cell injections seem to be best suited for fine lines with the current on-label indication of nasolabial wrinkle correction.
- Compared with hyaluronic acid and other inert fillers, additional costs for harvesting and culturing before injection are incurred.
- Side effects are minimal and comparable with other injected agents.

INTRODUCTION

Biologic aging of the skin, often accelerated by ultraviolet radiation, involves the loss of ground substance, hyaluronic acid (HA), subcutaneous fatty tissue, and collagen and elastic fibers. The age at which this degradation occurs depends on several factors including genetic predisposition, deleterious environmental factors, cigarette smoke exposure, and excessive alcohol consumption.

Unwanted wrinkles can be corrected using a variety of methods including lasers, both ablative and nonablative, a variety of soft tissue fillers, and botulinum toxin for dynamic rhytids. For fillers, the goal is to fill depressions but, at the same time, induce a biologic response that includes replacement of degraded components such as elastin, ground substance, and HA. A variety of fillers can be used but typically degradable or semipermanent or permanent dermal fillers are in use. Of

several types of products available, the most commonly used dermal filler is HA.

HAs can be extracted from animal tissue (eg, rooster combs) or produced using gene technology or fermentative processes from equine streptococcal strains not pathologic to humans. These chemically modified, cross-linked polymers are biologically inert, water insoluble, and more or less viscoelastic. To prevent the rapid degradation of HA and prolong its persistence in the skin, cross-linked HAs are injected into the dermis or subcutaneous tissue.

Unlike fillers, the newest therapy for rhytids consists of autologous cell injection. Cell injection is not a dermal filler, not stem cells (but may contain stem cells, which is under investigation), a synthetic product or foreign material, growth factors, or a cosmeceutical. Autologous fibroblasts are the first and only autologous fibroblast cell therapy approved by the US Food and Drug Administration (FDA) for aesthetic use that is

[a] Department of Dermatology, Johns Hopkins University School of Medicine, Baltimore, MD, USA; [b] The Maryland Laser, Skin, and Vein Institute, 54 Scott Adam Road, Hunt Valley, Baltimore, MD 21030, USA
* The Maryland Laser, Skin, and Vein Institute, 54 Scott Adam Road, Hunt Valley, Baltimore, MD 21030.
E-mail address: rweiss@smoothskin.net

Facial Plast Surg Clin N Am 21 (2013) 299–304
http://dx.doi.org/10.1016/j.fsc.2013.02.008
1064-7406/13/$ – see front matter © 2013 Published by Elsevier Inc.

grown from patient-specific biopsies and injected back into facial skin. This therapy most likely injects fibroblasts lost to aging and apoptosis, as well as diminished collagen. The goal is also to stimulate a biologic response that, in turn, triggers replacement of degraded components such as elastin, ground substance, and HA. With experience still at the early stages, it is possible that this cell therapy may replace superficial synthetic fillers, but currently that is doubtful. Autologous fibroblasts have a key role as a superficial filler that may be synergistic to volume fillers already used in clinical practice. Autologous fibroblasts also have possibilities to provide a long-term solution for increase of quality and quantity of dermal collagen bundles.

PIVOTAL STUDY FOR FDA CLEARANCE OF AUTOLOGOUS FIBROBLASTS

Clinical trials for autologous fibroblast therapy have been conducted since 2001. A major trial, reported in 2007, showed initial hopeful results.[1] This was a double-blind, randomized comparison of injectable living autologous fibroblast cells and placebo for the treatment of facial contour defects (N = 215). Live fibroblasts (20 million/mL) or placebo (the transport medium without living cells) were given as 3 doses administered at 1-week to 2-week intervals. Efficacy evaluations were performed 1, 2, 4, 6, 9, and 12 months after the first injection. Results indicated that living fibroblasts produced statistically significantly greater improvements in dermal deformities and acne scars than did placebo. The difference between live fibroblast injections and placebo achieved statistical significance at 6 months (P<.0001). At 9-month and 12-month follow-up, patients treated with live fibroblasts continued to show benefit from treatment with response rates of 75.0% and 81.6%, respectively. No serious treatment-related adverse events were reported. This finding led to the initial conclusion that autologous fibroblast injections could safely and effectively produce improvements in rhytids, acne scars, and other dermal defects continuing for at least 12 months after injection, providing the evidence that long-term improvement with cellular therapy was possible.

The current cellular therapy product called LAVIV (Fibrocell Science, Exton, PA) is the first cell therapy cleared by the FDA for aesthetic improvement and the first to show statistically significant benefit in large blinded controlled trials. This new category of cell therapy was subject to a more comprehensive study with clear end points for success than studies of most other aesthetic therapies currently provided. For clearance to treat in the United States, autologous fibroblast therapy required a parallel design, resulting in 2 large, well-powered studies that showed clinical benefit to a high degree of statistical significance.[2] Fibroblast injection was compared with placebo injection of a saline equivalent (transport medium for biopsies). The comparison was an intersubject design rather than previous trials that were intrasubject comparisons. Previous studies to treat the nasolabial fold (NLF) area were intrasubject designs in which the new treatment was compared with an existing bovine collagen injection on contralateral NLFs.[3–6]

The results of the pivotal study included data on 372 subjects. Seventy-eight percent of subjects treated with autologous fibroblast therapy and 48% of subjects treated with placebo achieved at least a 1-point improvement on the subject assessment at 6 months (P<.001), and 64% of subjects treated with autologous fibroblast therapy and 36% of those treated with placebo showed at least a 1-point improvement in the evaluator's assessment (P<.001). Adverse events were generally mild, and the treatment was well tolerated. Adverse events are listed in **Table 1**.

PREOPERATIVE: LOGISTICS OF OBTAINING BIOPSY AND SCHEDULING INJECTION

Once a patient is identified and has been informed, Fibrocell is contacted, following which a patient-specific biopsy shipper package is cataloged.

Table 1 Adverse events with autologous fibroblast therapy		
	LAVIV (508 Subjects) n (%)	Vehicle (354 Subjects) n (%)
Any injection site reaction	343 (67)	144 (40)
Erythema	81 (16)	33 (9)
Bruising	54 (11)	48 (14)
Swelling	69 (14)	15 (4)
Pain	31 (6)	6 (2)
Hemorrhage	13 (3)	16 (5)
Edema	22 (4)	0
Nodules	20 (4)	3 (<1)
Papules	8 (2)	3 (<1)
Irritation	6 (1)	1 (<1)
Dermatitis	5 (1)	2 (<1)
Pruritus	5 (1)	3 (<1)

The patient biopsy is then scheduled in advance by the practice, in conjunction with a Fibrocell representative, so that the laboratory will be able to receive and process the biopsy. Once scheduled, a personalized biopsy kit/shipper is sent to the practice location. This biopsy kit/shipper is specially designed to ship live biologics and includes biopsy packaging materials (ie, biopsy vial, Tyvek envelopes) that are prelabeled with the patient's initials, date of birth, personal identification number (PIN), and physician site code. It is important to remember that biopsies can be performed from Monday to Thursday so that, when shipped by FedEx, they can be processed for culture the next morning on Tuesday to Friday. In a similar way, when scheduling a patient for injection of cells, the FedEx shipment of cells from the laboratory can occur on Monday to Thursday for injection on Tuesday to Friday.

PROCEDURE: BIOPSY TECHNIQUE

Three 3-mm punch biopsies are performed in 1 retroauricular area to harvest donor fibroblasts (**Fig. 1**). If more than 3 are taken, only the best 3 are sent.

- The biopsies are performed all at 1 sitting, in the postauricular area, with just enough depth to obtain cells from the dermis, but not as deep as adipose tissue.
- If adipose tissue is obtained, the fat is trimmed before filling the vial.
- Blood or hair should be disposed of before placement of the 3 biopsies in the transport media vial.

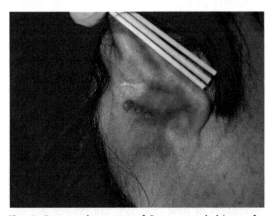

Fig. 1. Proper placement of 3-mm punch biopsy for harvest to culture fibroblasts. Full-thickness skin is required for dermal tissue. Tumescence with 1% lidocaine allows placement of biopsy within the postauricular fold. Once local anesthesia dissipates, these biopsy sites become oval to slits, allowing for rapid healing without sutures.

- All biopsies are submitted in single vials prelabeled with the patient's initials, date of birth, PIN, and physician site code.
- Donor sites are closed with sutures or adhesive bandages or left open to heal by secondary intention at the discretion of the physician.
- Donor material is processed as detailed later.

FIBROBLAST CULTURE

After biopsy collection, skin samples are placed in a vial and submerged in phosphate buffered saline (PBS), and shipped overnight at 2° to 8°C to the Fibrocell facility for processing. Once received at the sponsor facility, biopsy samples are inspected for quality and transferred to manufacturing for processing and tissue culture plating.

All cell processing occurs under aseptic conditions (ISO 5, 209E Class 100) within a biologic safety cabinet. Manufacturing activities occur under current good manufacturing practices. After an antibiotic wash containing gentamicin and amphotericin B, biopsy tissue is subjected to enzymatic dissociation in a collagenase enzyme cocktail at 37°C (Liberase Blendzyme, Roche, Penzberg, Germany).

Cells are then seeded into a T-175 culture flask within Iscove modified Dulbecco medium (IMDM) with phenol red supplemented with antibiotics and fetal bovine serum (FBS). Culture flasks are stored in a humidified incubator at 37°C with 5% carbon dioxide. Routine feeding of the fibroblasts is performed using IMDM with FBS by removing half of the volume of spent medium and adding back the volume with fresh medium. Once the culture reaches confluence specifications, cells are rinsed with PBS and exposed to trypsin–ethylenediaminetetraacetic acid to remove cells from the surface of the flask. Cells are then transferred to a T-500 triple culture flask. After confluence is achieved in the T-500 flask, cells are rinsed and transferred, using trypsinization, into a 10-layer cell stack. After reconfluence in this cell stack, fibroblasts are harvested and cryopreserved in IMDM and freezing medium (Profreeze, Lonza, Walkersville, MD) supplemented with dimethyl sulfoxide. Cells are stored in the vapor phase of liquid nitrogen. After cryopreservation, addition series of release tests are performed, including efficacy analyses confirming the cell population count, 85% or greater viability, and identity of the overall population as 98% or more fibroblasts.

Before use, the cells are thawed, washed with PBS and Dulbecco Modified Eagle Medium,

resuspended at a concentration of 1.0 to 2.0 ×
107 cells/mL, and shipped overnight at 2° to 8°C
to the treatment center for administration the
next day. Before shipment, a series of additional
efficacy release tests are performed on the final
product, including confirmation of cell count and
assessment of cell viability. In addition, safety
tests, including Gram stain, endotoxin detection,
and sterility, are performed on each released injection set in the series. Before use at the treatment
center, the cell suspension is stored at 2° to 8°C
and then allowed to warm to room temperature
for 30 minutes before use.

PROCEDURE: CELL INJECTION TECHNIQUE

- Anesthesia may be topical, local infiltrative,
  or regional blocks using customary local
  anesthetic agents. Typically, only topical
  anesthetic is used.
- The area of treatment is prepared with
  cleansing by alcohol just before injections
  with time allowed for the alcohol to
  evaporate.
- After gentle inversion of the vial to dislodge
  clumped cells, aspiration into a 1-mL or
  3-mL syringe is performed using a 22-gauge
  to 25-gauge needle.
- The cell suspension is injected using
  30-gauge needle in a retrograde threading
  technique or in small aliquots of 0.05 to
  0.1 mL directly into a wrinkle.

Injection note: no lidocaine or epinephrine is
added to the cell suspension before injection
because of the negative impact on the viability of
the cells.

- The injection is into the superficial papillary
  dermis and confirmed by the appearance of
  blanching and wheal formation at the site of
  each injection (**Fig. 2**).

Injection note: no massage or other manipulation of the areas is performed to avoid risk of
damaging or altering the cells.

- Subjects are advised to avoid the use of
  soaps, cosmetics, or any other products to
  the face for 72 hours after each injection
  session, although mild washing is permitted.
  After injections, indirect application of ice to
  the treatment area is permitted but not
  recommended.

The current treatment regimen of 3 administration sessions, each 5 weeks apart, with
a dose of 0.1 mL of a suspension of 1.0 to 2.0 ×
107 cells/mL is ideal.

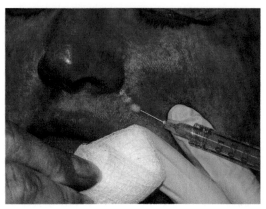

Fig. 2. Proper injection technique. The injection is
into the superficial papillary dermis and confirmed
by the appearance of blanching and wheal formation
at the site of each injection. A threading technique
may be used but serial puncture is most commonly
used, as shown here.

MECHANISM OF ACTION OF INJECTED AUTOLOGOUS FIBROBLASTS

Prior studies focused on multiple facial areas and
ideal dosing concentrations and frequencies. The
exact mechanism of action of injected autologous
fibroblasts remains unknown. They may exert their
effect through one of several mechanisms that
could include the direct synthesis of increased
amounts of collagen and elastin, the induced
proliferation of native fibroblasts, or the deposition
of cofactors or increase in population of fibroblasts.[7] A study of the histologic changes including tissue responses and adverse reactions
in skin treated with autologous fibroblasts at
3 months postinjection has shown that cellular
morphology in the dermis shows no abnormalities
along with no changes in quality of matrix, quality
of collagen/elastin, or epidermal/dermal thickness
between adjacent control skin and forearm skin
injected with autologous fibroblasts (data on file,
Fibrocell Science, Exton, PA).

OUTCOMES: DURATION OF EFFECT OF CELL INJECTION

The timeline for wrinkle improvement with autologous fibroblasts is unlike that of most dermal
fillers. Autologous cells most likely increase the
deposition of new collagen, but do not act like
a volumizer filler. There is a more gradual onset
of action than the immediate correction seen
with HA dermal fillers.

Clinical improvement in NLF wrinkles were seen
as early as 2 months after the start of treatment
and before the injection series was completed,

with continuous improvement seen in the follow-up months 2 to 6 after a series of 3 injections.[2] Unlike most dermal filler products, autologous fibroblast therapy benefit is not expected to degrade over 6 months.[8,9] Prior studies of autologous fibroblasts showed continued benefit 1 year after treatment.[1] The duration of effect is not known. Anecdotal evidence suggests that some patients treated in clinical trials 8 years ago still show clinical benefit for NLF (R Weiss, 2012, personal observation).

The FDA-cleared indication is for treatment of NLF wrinkles. The improvement seen is in wrinkles, not volume filling of deep folds. Other potential indications include but are not limited to glabella folds, periocular rhytids, tear troughs, upper lip rhytids, marionette lines, chest wrinkles, necklace lines, atrophic skin of the dorsal hands, acne scars, surgical scars, and burn scars (**Fig. 3**). Clinical trials are currently underway for acne and burn scars.

Summary of fillers versus autologous therapy					
Therapy	Immediate	2 mo	2–6 mo	>6 mo	1 y
Autologous fibroblast injection	No change	1 injection: nasolabial fold wrinkles improved	3 injections: continuous improvement in wrinkles	No degradation of filler	Continued benefit
HA dermal filler	Wrinkles corrected			Filler degradation	Additional injection

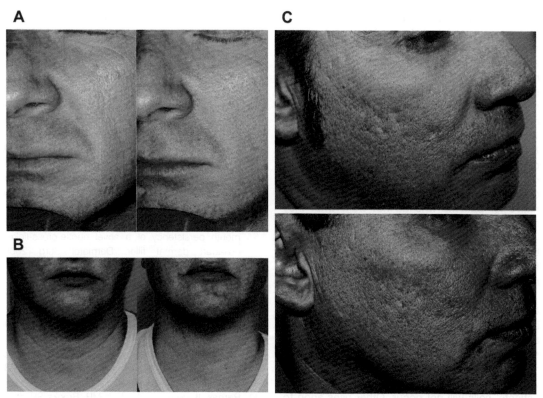

Fig. 3. Clinical effect of autologous fibroblast injection. Indicated use in NLF wrinkles shows (*A*) before (*left*) and after (*right*) 12 months. Clinically significant effect is noted by both patient and treating physician. (*B*) Off-label use for necklace lines; before treatment (the control) is shown on the left, whereas 1 month after the second treatment of the right side to neck midline shows significant improvement on the right. (*C*) Treatment of acne scarring shows significant improvement of injected scars at 1 year after a series of 3 injections 2 weeks apart.

SIDE EFFECTS OF AUTOLOGOUS FIBROBLAST THERAPY

Adverse events as listed in **Table 1** indicate that autologous fibroblast therapy treatments are as safe as many of the existing filler therapies.[10] The local findings of erythema, bruising, and swelling in the treatment area are expected and have a short overall duration. No hypersensitivity reactions were noted, and no long-term nodules or other local problems were seen. A theoretic risk of the enhancement of malignancies with autologous cell therapy has been raised.[11] Although 1 basal cell carcinoma was reported near a treatment site in the pivotal trial, it is unrelated to the autologous fibroblast injection for 2 reasons:

1. Given the number of subjects and duration of the trial, the incidence of cutaneous malignancy is consistent with background rates.
2. Basal cell carcinoma is not a fibroblast-derived tumor. To date, no dermatofibro sarcomas have been reported in thousands of injections.

SUMMARY

Cultured autologous fibroblasts seem to be the first successful implementation of a new FDA-cleared class designated as cell therapy for treatment of wrinkles. Unlike conventional fillers, cells are injected more superficially and may require months to show improvement. Patients must be informed that cell therapy does not work immediately. Autologous cells provide gradual improvement after 3 serial treatments over several weeks. This treatment offers the promise of sustained growth of living cells that may have greater persistence than other fillers, although follow-up in routine clinical use has not yet been shown. Autologous fibroblast cell injection may be a good alternative for patients who do not want what they perceive to be extraneous or foreign materials injected. Fibroblasts are not a volume filler; fibroblast cell injections seem to be best suited for fine lines with the current on-label indication of nasolabial wrinkle correction.

Compared with HA and other inert fillers, additional costs for harvesting and culturing before injection are incurred. Side effects are minimal and comparable with other injected agents. A strict protocol in which a PIN number is assigned, associated with a patient's birthday and initials, virtually ensures that the inadvertent mix-up of patients' cells will not occur. Other uses soon to be considered by the FDA for marketing include autologous fibroblasts for acne scars and burn scars. Some physicians are currently using the product for off-label indications of wrinkles on other parts of the face and other body areas. Long-term results are expected, but not proved.

REFERENCES

1. Weiss RA, Weiss MA, Beasley KL, et al. Autologous cultured fibroblast injection for facial contour deformities: a prospective, placebo-controlled, phase III clinical trial. Dermatol Surg 2007;33(3):263–8.
2. Smith SR, Munavalli G, Weiss R, et al. A multicenter, double-blind, placebo-controlled trial of autologous fibroblast therapy for the treatment of nasolabial fold wrinkles. Dermatol Surg 2012;38(7 Pt 2): 1234–43.
3. Narins RS, Brandt F, Leyden J, et al. A randomized, double-blind, multicenter comparison of the efficacy and tolerability of Restylane versus Zyplast for the correction of nasolabial folds. Dermatol Surg 2003; 29(6):588–95.
4. Brandt FS, Cazzaniga A, Baumann L, et al. Investigator global evaluations of efficacy of injectable poly-L-lactic acid versus human collagen in the correction of nasolabial fold wrinkles. Aesthet Surg J 2011;31(5):521–8.
5. Carruthers A, Carey W, De Lorenzi C, et al. Randomized, double-blind comparison of the efficacy of two hyaluronic acid derivatives, Restylane Perlane and Hylaform, in the treatment of nasolabial folds. Dermatol Surg 2005;31(11 Pt 2):1591–8 [discussion: 1598].
6. Baumann LS, Shamban AT, Lupo MP, et al. Comparison of smooth-gel hyaluronic acid dermal fillers with cross-linked bovine collagen: a multicenter, double-masked, randomized, within-subject study. Dermatol Surg 2007;33(Suppl 2):S128–35.
7. Lamme EN, Van Leeuwen RT, Brandsma K, et al. Higher numbers of autologous fibroblasts in an artificial dermal substitute improve tissue regeneration and modulate scar tissue formation. J Pathol 2000; 190(5):595–603.
8. Narins RS, Brandt FS, Lorenc ZP, et al. Twelve-month persistency of a novel ribose-cross-linked collagen dermal filler. Dermatol Surg 2008; 34(Suppl 1):S31–9.
9. Smith SR, Jones D, Thomas JA, et al. Duration of wrinkle correction following repeat treatment with Juvederm hyaluronic acid fillers. Arch Dermatol Res 2010;302(10):757–62 PubMed Central PMCID: 2970825.
10. Cohen JL. Understanding, avoiding, and managing dermal filler complications. Dermatol Surg 2008; 34(Suppl 1):S92–9.
11. Barnas JL, Simpson-Abelson MR, Brooks SP, et al. Reciprocal functional modulation of the activation of T lymphocytes and fibroblasts derived from human solid tumors. J Immunol 2010;185(5): 2681–92.

Index

Note: Page numbers of article titles are in **boldface** type.

Moving?

Make sure your subscription moves with you!

To notify us of your new address, find your **Clinics Account Number** (located on your mailing label above your name), and contact customer service at:

Email: journalscustomerservice-usa@elsevier.com

800-654-2452 (subscribers in the U.S. & Canada)
314-447-8871 (subscribers outside of the U.S. & Canada)

Fax number: 314-447-8029

Elsevier Health Sciences Division
Subscription Customer Service
3251 Riverport Lane
Maryland Heights, MO 63043

*To ensure uninterrupted delivery of your subscription, please notify us at least 4 weeks in advance of move.

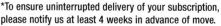

ELSEVIER

Printed and bound by CPI Group (UK) Ltd, Croydon, CR0 4YY

03/10/2024

01040332-0012